Infertility
Finding God's Peace in the Journey

Lois Flowers

HARVEST HOUSE™ PUBLISHERS

EUGENE, OREGON

Cover by Koechel Peterson & Associates, Inc., Minneapolis, Minnesota

Author photo on back cover by Scott Flanagin

INFERTILITY—FINDING GOD'S PEACE IN THE JOURNEY
Copyright © 2003 by Lois Flowers
Published by Harvest House Publishers
Eugene, Oregon 97402

Library of Congress Cataloging-in-Publication Data
 Flowers, Lois, 1970–
  Infertility: finding God's peace in the journey / Lois Flowers.
   p. cm.
 Includes bibliographical references.
  ISBN 0-7369-1180-4 (pbk.)
  1. Infertility—Religious aspects—Christianity. 2. Consolation. I. Title.
  RC889.F56 2003
  248.8'6196692—dc21   2003001829

Printed in the United States of America

03   04   05   06   07   08   09   10   / BP - CF /   10   9   8   7   6   5   4   3   2   1

"Is there life during infertility? Lois Flowers believes that there is, and using stories from her own journey backed up by solid biblical truth, she shows her readers how they can experience it. *Infertility—Finding God's Peace in the Journey* will transform the way you look at your infertility, your future, and your relationship with God."

—Greg T. Smalley, PsyD
President/CEO of Smalley Relationship Center

"Moving, authentic, and powerful—a must-read for any couple experiencing the painful process of infertility. You will laugh out loud and tears will flow freely as you journey with Lois and her husband through their story of infertility. Woven throughout each chapter is the very practical application of God's Word that they gleaned along the way. A true inspiration and encouragement you will not soon forget!"

—Deene Hyde,
adoptive mother, pastor's wife,
and Women's Ministry Bible Study Teacher,
First Baptist Church of Springdale, Arkansas

"Not only is this resource filled with practical help and hope, it is very readable as well as biblically insightful. Anyone struggling with this issue will be thankful that the author took the time to share from her life and heart."

—Dr. H. Norman Wright,
nationally known marriage and family counselor
and bestselling author of more than 65 books,
including Quiet Times for Couples

"As someone who also traveled the journey of infertility, I found Lois Flowers' experience strikingly familiar in some ways and utterly unique in others—but it's her transparency that makes this book authentic. Not only does Lois let us see how she and her husband, Randy, managed to find God's peace amid uncertainty, but she gives us a whole range of tools to deal with disappointment, medical trauma, and insensitive, inquisitive people. This book will resonate with those who are fellow travelers on this journey."

—Wendy Lawton,
author, adoptive mother, founder and
president of the Lawton Doll Company

To Randy—
because this isn't just my story.

Acknowledgments

Many thanks—

—to the other writers who challenged and inspired me as I was writing this book, including Philip Yancey, C.S. Lewis, Michael R. Phillips, and Charles Swindoll.

—to Joy DeKok, Karen Hopkins, Deene Hyde, Lea Ellen Jones, Mary McCully, Debbie Pschierer, Esther Ware, and Tricia Withers for reviewing the manuscript and offering valuable feedback.

—to Dr. Gary Oliver, for believing in this project.

—to all the wonderful folks at Harvest House, especially LaRae Weikert and Paul Gossard, for helping my dream for this book to become reality.

—to Nancy Caver Jeffery, who, perhaps more than anyone besides my husband, helped me plow through my thoughts and figure out what God has been teaching me during the last five years.

—to my sister and brother-in-law, Ruth and Jerry Keehner, for your passionate belief in the message of this book and in my ability to deliver it.

—to my mom, Angela Reimers, for your constant encouragement, and to my dad, Robert Reimers, for teaching me how to think.

—to all our other friends and family members who prayed for us as we waited for God to unfold His plan for our family.

—to my husband, Randy, for loving me and taking care of me.

Finally, I offer praise and thanksgiving to my Lord and Savior Jesus Christ, "the Father of compassion and the God of all comfort, who comforts us in all our troubles, so that we can comfort those in any trouble with the comfort we ourselves have received from God" (2 Corinthians 1:3-4).

Contents

Hope in the Midst of Heartache

A Note from Gary and Carrie Oliver

Did you know that one in ten Americans of childbearing age has fertility problems? Did you know that infertility affects 9 million American couples every year?

That's okay—we didn't either.

It's been more than 20 years since I (Gary) saw my first couple struggling with infertility. I knew very little about it, and there were few resources for a young therapist to turn to. I didn't understand the complexity of all of the issues involved. I didn't understand the relentless physical, emotional, and financial stress a couple experiences. I had no idea what it was like to wade through the emotional, ethical, and financial complications of the reproductive options that were then becoming available.

As with many others, my initial thought was that infertility was primarily a medical issue. But as Lois so clearly points out, "A medical issue regarding infertility—whether it has to do with ovulation irregularities, blocked tubes, endometriosis, multiple miscarriages, low sperm counts, incorrect hormone levels, or anything else—is never just a medical issue. It comes with a whole host of emotional and spiritual ramifications. Some of these can be resolved fairly quickly, but others bring a fresh onslaught of distress that may never go away completely."

I wish I'd understood that 20 years ago.

We never struggled with infertility, but we've worked with hundreds of couples who have—and we wish we'd had this book to recommend years ago. What Lois has written is stimulating, informative, challenging, and refreshing. Here you'll find no shallow, superficial, pie-in-the-sky platitudes or an invitation to a self-serving pity party. Lois asks and answers the hard questions…and the heart questions. Though she isn't a psychologist, she thinks and writes with a psychological sensitivity. Though she's not a trained Bible scholar, she thinks and writes biblically.

This book will give you a fresh perspective on what mercy and grace look like. You'll discover that in the midst of heartache you can find hope. In the midst of hopelessness and the sense that you are all alone, you can experience being ambushed by God's grace. In the midst of walking through an emotional minefield, you can find a peace that passes all understanding. (And the helpful appendix for friends and family members is an added bonus. It alone is worth the price of the book.)

This book has a happy ending. Not because Lois and her husband, Randy, were finally able to conceive, but for what they allowed God to *show* them and how they allowed God to *grow* them through the process. Over the years we've discovered that God doesn't always answer our prayers like we want Him to. But He does always answer them. His grace is sufficient. His mercies are new every morning.

—Gary and Carrie Oliver

Gary J. Oliver, PhD, is executive director of The Center for Marriage & Family Studies (CMFS) and Professor of Psychology and Practical Theology at John Brown University. Carrie Oliver, MA, is a counselor specializing in marriage, family, and women's issues, a conference speaker and, with Gary, co-author of Raising Sons and Loving It!

My Pile of Stones

❦

$\mathcal{I}$n Old Testament times, when an individual or a group of people witnessed a miraculous act of God or had a personal encounter with Him, they often erected a stone or a pile of stones as a memorial to what they had seen and heard.

The patriarch Jacob did it the morning after God appeared to him in a dream and told him that his descendants would become a great nation (Genesis 28:10-19). The Israelites did it after they crossed the Jordan River on dry ground into the promised land (Joshua 3:14–4:9). And the prophet Samuel did it after God routed the Philistine army on behalf of the nation of Israel (1 Samuel 7:10-13).

These monuments were signs—to the people who erected them and to their descendants—of God's faithfulness and power. Whenever they passed by them, they were reminded of what He had done for them and among them at that time. The stones were a tangible testimonial that the God who had been faithful and true in the past would remain faithful and true forever.

This book is my pile of stones.

It is a memorial to the infertility journey that God has led me and my husband, Randy, on over the last several years. This journey has not always been easy—in fact, it has been marked by pain, sadness, and disappointment. But along the way, those feelings have been tempered by peace and a growing sense of joy.

In case you're wondering, God has not chosen—at least not thus far—to remove the thorn of infertility from our side. We haven't had that perfect ending that many childless couples long for—a positive pregnancy test that results in a happy, healthy newborn. But as we navigated the waters of infertility together, Randy and I developed an acute sense of God's hand on our lives. It didn't come overnight, of course, but as we watched God move in one seemingly coincidental way after another, we came to realize that, although our family life wasn't progressing in the way we thought and hoped it would, it was progressing in the way *He* wanted it to progress.

God didn't always answer our prayers like we wanted Him to answer them. But He did answer them.

Sometimes He said yes. Many times He said no. But most often, He seemed to answer with a simple, deeply probing question: *Do you trust Me? Do you trust Me to handle the future of your family? Do you trust Me to know what I'm doing with your life? When you want to do it your way, when you start doubting My faithfulness, when you start comparing yourself to others…do you trust Me?*

As we pondered these difficult questions, we came to realize that ultimately, our answers had much more to do with the way we viewed God and how He related to us as His children than they did with our desire to bring our own child into the world. Did we really believe all the things we had been taught about God for so many years—that He loves us, that He knows what's best for us, that He hears and answers our prayers, that He is in control of *everything*? Or did we embrace our faith in a sovereign God only when it was easy or convenient for us? It wasn't a dramatic crisis of belief, but it was a crisis of belief nonetheless, one that quietly confronted us time and time again.

What was God up to in our lives? Why were we unable to conceive the baby we longed for when people around us were getting pregnant without even trying? What was the point to all of this?

As we sat in waiting rooms, endured emotional and physical pain, braved surgeries, and navigated the monthly cycle of hope followed by disappointment, we clung to God's promise in Romans 8:28: "We know that in all things God works for the good of those who love him, who have been called according to his purpose."

"Lord," we prayed, "don't let our sadness, our disappointment, and our pain be for nothing. If we have to go through this, *please* let us use our experiences to touch others."

That's why I'm writing this book.

I'm not a physician. I'm not a marriage and family counselor. I'm not a theologian. I'm certainly not a super-Christian with an unusually large amount of faith. Far from it, in fact. I'm simply a person whose life has been profoundly altered by my experience

---

*W*hy *were we unable to conceive the baby we longed for when people around us were getting pregnant without even trying?*

---

with infertility. It has affected my health, my family, my marriage, my attitude toward the suffering of others, my interactions with friends, my prayer life, and—most importantly—my relationship with God. Having been so affected, I feel compelled to share bits and pieces from my journey in hopes that they might help someone else who is facing the same kind of trial.

You may not agree with all the conclusions I've come to. Your infertility journey may have taken you down roads I've never traveled. You may have a different take on faith, on prayer, on coping, or on options for medical treatment. That's all fine with me. My intent is not to tell you how to think, what decisions you should make, or how you should feel. I simply want to present a perspective on dealing with infertility that you may not get from your doctor, your well-meaning friends and loved ones, or even your church.

Most of us don't plan to be infertile. We believe that child-bearing is a normal and cherished part of family life, and we just assume we'll get pregnant when we're ready. So when things don't go according to our plan, our whole world is thrown into a tizzy, and understandably so. For some reason, perhaps because God created us with an innate desire to create and nurture, the inability to have a baby often seems to pose greater challenges to our faith and emotions than other difficult trials we might encounter in our lives. We've been taught all our lives that children are a blessing from the Lord—so why wouldn't He want us to enjoy His blessings like everyone else around us?

That, my friend, is the $64,000 question. I don't have all the answers, but I hope that the principles that have helped Randy and me deal with our own infertility problems will comfort your heart, strengthen your faith, and bolster your confidence that God has a special plan for *your* life.

Finding Peace Along the Way

Every month, as I endure varying amounts of physical pain stemming from the condition that caused my infertility, I'm reminded of the fact that I probably never will get pregnant. The fact that, as I write, my husband and I are in the process of adopting a little girl from China means that we are no longer trying to conceive, but it does not change the fact that I am—as the Scriptures so bluntly put it—*barren*.

Even now, writing that word isn't easy. In fact, I really don't like it one bit. But despite the occasional bouts with sadness and unexpected surges of emotion that I still feel every now and then, despite my ongoing physical problems, and despite the questions that may forever go unresolved, I've learned to accept the path my life has taken. I can't say I wake up every morning and thank God for my infertility, but I can say, without hesitation, that I do thank Him for the growth that has occurred in my life as a result of it.

I don't know where you are today in your efforts to conceive. Maybe you're just starting out—but because you have several friends who have had infertility problems, you wonder if you might have them too. Maybe, after trying to get pregnant for a year or so, you're starting to suspect that something is wrong, and you're not quite sure what to make of it. Perhaps you've just had your first visit with an infertility specialist and you're completely overwhelmed by all the treatment options.

Maybe you're perplexed by all the ethical questions associated with assisted reproductive techniques and find that your doctor isn't willing to address your concerns. Maybe you're waiting to find out if a costly procedure was successful, or perhaps you've just realized the crushing truth that one was not. Maybe you've even experienced the joy of a positive pregnancy test and the first few months of "expecting," only to have your heart broken and hopes dashed by a painful miscarriage.

Maybe, after years of disappointment and heartache, you're thinking about putting an end to all the infertility treatments, but you're afraid that calling it quits somehow displays a lack of faith. Or maybe you gave up trying to get pregnant years ago, but you still find yourself grieving the loss of your dream every now and then.

Whatever your situation, this book is for you.

Before you dive in, let me tell you what you will not find in these pages. You won't find detailed information about the pros and cons of all the various treatment options and infertility procedures your doctor might want you to consider. Nor will you find dozens of testimonials designed to help you realize you're not alone in your struggles with infertility. Other books, some written from a Christian perspective, cover those things very well.

You also won't find a great deal of emphasis on infertility "success" stories, from Scripture or from anywhere else. By not focusing on Sarah, Rachel, Hannah, Elizabeth, and other women of the Bible who were barren and then conceived, I don't mean to imply that their experiences don't apply to us or that they cannot be of some encouragement to us. Nor do I want to discourage anyone who truly desires to become pregnant. I do recognize, however, that although some of the people who read this book will conceive and go on to give birth to a healthy child, others will not. That's why this book is as much about learning to accept God's path for your life—particularly when that path may not allow you to realize dreams that have long been dear to your heart—as it is about adopting and maintaining a healthy spiritual perspective as you try to have a baby.

You may wonder if, as the title of this book suggests, it's really possible to find God's peace through the journey of infertility. Please believe me when I say that it is. Philippians 4:6-7 says, "Do not be anxious about anything, but in everything, by prayer and petition, with thanksgiving, present your requests to God. *And the peace of God, which transcends all understanding, will guard your hearts and your minds in Christ Jesus.*"

God's peace is deep. It's abiding. During the battles of infertility, it provides a protective covering for our emotions, our hearts, and our souls. I know, because it has protected me.

That peace may be eluding you right now. In fact, you may wonder if you'll ever experience it. I know that you can. I hope that you will. And I pray that this book, in some small way, will help illuminate the way for you.

Lamentations 3:22-26, a biblical anchor for me when Randy and I were trying to conceive, declares,

> *Because of the* LORD's *great love we are not consumed,*
> *for his compassions never fail.*
> *They are new every morning;*
> *great is your faithfulness.*
> *I say to myself, "The* LORD *is my portion;*
> *therefore I will wait for him."*
> *The* LORD *is good to those whose hope is in him,*
> *to the one who seeks him;*
> *it is good to wait quietly*
> *for the salvation of the* LORD.

The process of erecting my pile of stones—in book form—is a vivid reminder of all the quiet waiting that we did. But it also brings to mind all those times when we felt the arms of our loving heavenly Father securely wrapped around us, constantly reassuring us that no matter what we wanted, He was all we really needed.

The Lord *is* good to those whose hope is in Him. Remember that as you wait.

ONE

Why Peace Is Elusive

⌘

*M*y earliest career aspiration was a simple one: When I grew up, I wanted to be a mother.

This goal probably had something to do with the fact that, for the first five years of my life, my primary female role model was my own mom, a stay-at-home wife and mother whose chief occupation in life was caring for me, my five older siblings, and my father. From my perspective as a little girl, being a mother was an extremely important job. No one else could cook supper, shop for groceries, buy those all-important Christmas and birthday presents, bundle me up to play in the snow, kiss scraped knees, or make chocolate-chip cookies any better.

When I was five, I accompanied my dad to the hospital to bring home my mom and my new baby sister. I remember sitting in the backseat of my dad's 1969 Rambler, stretching to get a glimpse of the little bundle in my mom's arms. I didn't know about all the responsibility and heartache that goes with parenthood—I just knew I wanted to be a mom.

As I grew older, my ambitions gradually changed. After I started school, I wanted to be a teacher; then, a contemporary

Christian singer; and finally, a businesswoman who wore classy suits, lived in a trendy apartment, and carried a briefcase to work every day. Along the way—once I figured out what giving birth actually entailed—I set my maternal aspirations on a shelf where they were out of sight, yet still reachable. I planned to have several children when I got married, but there was no sense thinking about the terrifying mechanics of childbirth until that was absolutely necessary.

Fast-forward to May 1993. A few weeks after I graduated from college (with a degree in journalism—not business, music, or elementary education), I had major abdominal surgery to remove a grapefruit-sized cyst on one of my ovaries. I had always been healthy, and before this procedure, I had had no reason to think I had any of the "female" problems that plagued other women my age. I just assumed this surgery would be a one-time thing—that the doctor would fix me and I'd be as good as new from then on.

I was wrong.

When the doctor opened me up, he discovered that the cyst was only part of the problem. On top of that, a severe case of stage 4 endometriosis had frozen my bowels and reproductive organs into one stiff mass. The doctor did his best to eliminate the endometriosis, as well as the scar tissue and adhesions that caused all my organs to stick together, but he was unable to remove it all. After the surgery was over, he told my mother and Randy (who was then my boyfriend) that the severity of my condition would probably make it very difficult for me ever to get pregnant. In my muddled postoperative state, I just remember him saying that when the time came for me to try to conceive, I would likely need to have laparoscopic surgery first.

I didn't realize it at the time, but that surgery was the beginning of our infertility journey.

Randy and I were married in March 1994. We devoted our first few years as husband and wife to strengthening our already close relationship and working to pay off school bills. The doctor's evaluation of my fertility prospects notwithstanding, we didn't want any surprise pregnancies to interfere with our aggressive plan to repay our loans, so we were especially careful with my birth-control pills. Our caution seems a bit silly now, but even then I really didn't believe I'd have trouble getting pregnant. My mom had given birth to seven children, as had my maternal grandmother. Why would I be any different?

About three-and-a-half years after we got married, we decided we were ready to have a baby. Our school loans were paid off. We were building a new home. We were secure and happy in our marriage. The time was right. I began envisioning the perfect combination of our genes: a happy little girl with my wavy brown hair and Randy's clear blue eyes, or a cute little boy with Randy's penchant for woodworking and my love of books.

As we waited a few months for the birth-control pills to work themselves out of my system, I remember feeling very hopeful about our prospects. I hadn't forgotten what the doctor had said, but maybe—just maybe—he was wrong. *Wouldn't it be neat if I got pregnant right away?* I thought. *Wouldn't that be a real testament to God's power? He would definitely receive all the glory for performing such a miracle.* (Looking back, I realize rather sheepishly that those musings were only the first in a long line of such thoughts—as if I knew better than God what He should do to receive glory in my life.)

It didn't take long for that rosy color to fade off my glasses. As a year passed and my periods became more and more painful, I began to realize that the endometriosis I had pushed to the back of my mind for the last few years was making its ugly presence known once again. When my doctor heard that my pain felt very much like knives cutting into my lower abdomen, he scheduled a diagnostic laparoscopy.

The surgery was short. The endometriosis was so bad that all the doctor could do was remove a bit here and there and refer me to a specialist. "Don't even bother trying to get pregnant until you get that fixed," he told us. "It's not going to happen."

That was the beginning of a long series of doctor visits and uncomfortable procedures, including two more major surgeries. The first of those two surgeries supposedly removed all the endometriosis and greatly improved my chances of getting pregnant. Unfortunately, it failed to eliminate my most serious problem—the endometriosis that had invaded my colon. If left untreated, it could have caused a serious blockage in my bowel, which would have been far worse for my health than anything that might have been wrong with my reproductive system. So, eight months later—even before my body had had a chance to fully recover from the previous surgery—I was back in the hospital.

I went home six days later, leaving nearly eight inches of my colon and most of my dreams of ever becoming a mother in the usual way. In eight months' time, the endometriosis had all grown back. Once again, scar tissue and adhesions held my fallopian tubes and ovaries in place, preventing the mobility necessary for conception to occur. We could try to get pregnant on our own or by doing some minor fertility procedures, the doctor said, but given the aggressive nature of my disease, our only real chance at conceiving would be through in vitro fertilization (IVF).

That prognosis might seem to make our next step seem rather obvious. It wasn't.

Facing the Issues

Until now, I've described the basic physical facts of our infertility problems: I have this condition, this is what's been done to fix it, and these were the results. As a logical, practical person who has always been more of a thinker than a feeler, I would prefer to stop right there.

With infertility, that's impossible. A medical issue regarding fertility—whether it has to do with ovulation irregularities, blocked tubes, endometriosis, multiple miscarriages, low sperm counts, incorrect hormone levels, or anything else—is never just a medical issue. It comes with a whole host of emotional and spiritual ramifications. Some of these can be resolved fairly quickly, but others bring a fresh onslaught of distress that may never go away completely.

My mother had given birth to seven children, as had my maternal grandmother. Why would I be any different?

It's difficult for someone who has never experienced infertility to understand exactly how a woman who is having trouble conceiving feels about her body. We all have things that are wrong with us. Some of us are blind as a bat without corrected vision, some can't hear very well, some have high cholesterol or hypoglycemia, some have diabetes, some are overweight, some have asthma, and so on. For some reason, however, dealing with infertility is infinitely more difficult—more personally painful—than getting fitted for glasses, counting calories, or taking cholesterol-lowering medication. For whatever reason, poor vision, high cholesterol, and a host of other conditions—some which are directly caused by poor lifestyle choices—simply do not have the social stigma of infertility.

It's only in hindsight that I realize how Randy and I were affected by this stigma. Medically, a person is said to be infertile when conception fails to occur after a year of unprotected, well-timed intercourse. For us, that year passed before we even started any serious medical intervention. Technically, then, we were classified as infertile before my first laparoscopic surgery. In our minds, however, my problem wasn't infertility. Rather, it was endometriosis—an explainable medical problem that was easily corrected. Other people were infertile, not us.

Maybe it was denial. Maybe it was fear. Or maybe it was simply an unwillingness to acknowledge that we were among the 1 in 10 Americans of childbearing age who have fertility problems.[1] It was bad enough to be viewed as "that girl with endometriosis." The thought of being pitied for our inability to have children was intolerable.

Gradually, though, we began to realize that my endometriosis wasn't as correctable as we had originally hoped. Whether we liked it or not, infertility, still a bad word to both of us, was forcing its way into our vocabulary.

Facing the Feelings

During this time, there was one thought that kept occurring to me. No matter what the doctors did, there were parts of me that just didn't work like they were supposed to work. In a culture that depends on the efficiency and productivity of well-oiled machinery, we have a word for things like that—we call them broken. And that is exactly how I felt.

One night, I found something in Scripture that crystallized these feelings. I was lying on the floor reading my Bible when all of a sudden a verse from Psalm 31 flashed at me like a spotlight on a dark stage. "I have been ignored as if I were dead, as if I were a broken pot" (verse 12, NLT). I stopped, amazed at what I had just read.

"As if I were a broken pot."

I couldn't believe it! There, right in the middle of the Bible, was the perfect description of how I had felt so many times. My eyes quickly scanned the previous verses to see whether any of them applied as well. Though originally written by David, they too could have flowed just as easily from the pen of an infertile woman at the height of her despair!

> *Have mercy on me, LORD, for I am in distress*
>   *My sight is blurred because of my tears.*
>   *My body and soul are withering away.*
> *I am dying from grief;*
>   *my years are shortened by sadness.*
> *Misery has drained away my strength;*
>   *I am wasting from within.*
> *I am scorned by all my enemies*
>   *and even despised by my neighbors—*
>   *even my friends are afraid to come near me.*
> *When they see me on the street,*
>   *they turn the other way.*
> *I have been ignored as if I were dead,*
>   *as if I were a broken pot.*
>
> *—Psalm 31:9-12, NLT*

Those four verses capture the very essence of what goes on in your heart and mind when you're battling infertility. Each month that passes without a missed period saps a little bit more of your strength and makes a little bit more of your soul "wither away." Tears are always close by. You feel like an outcast, a misfit, a charter member of a club you never would have joined on your own.

Peace in the midst of that? It doesn't take a doctorate in psychology to see why it's often elusive.

Loss of Control

Before I go any further, I should point out that it's entirely possible to be at peace and still experience feelings of sadness, disappointment, frustration, and loneliness. The peace that I talk about in this book is not the absence of these difficult emotions.

Rather, it is the felt presence of something—of Someone—bigger than those feelings.

That said, for me, a lack of peace is characterized by worry, a knot in the pit of my stomach, or an unsettled feeling that just won't go away. For you, it might be tightness at the base of your neck, recurring headaches, sleeplessness, or some other physiological symptom. Whatever the case, when peace is gone, you know it.

The exact cause of the lack of peace might be a little harder to pin down. Any number of factors can play a role, and the effects of these factors vary from person to person depending on life experiences, spiritual background, and personality. They also vary throughout the infertility process. What might be a huge issue early in the journey might be entirely forgotten later, and vice versa.

For example, uneasiness about money was one of my earliest peace robbers. Our health insurance doesn't cover infertility-related expenses, and my greatest fear was that the insurance company would figure out I was trying to get pregnant and refuse to pay for the treatment I was getting for endometriosis. Medically, they were two separate issues. The endometriosis was a serious problem—even without my desire to conceive, it had to be corrected. But that didn't make me feel any better. I still worried about it. A lot.

One look at an infertility specialist's rate sheet is enough to produce a knot in the pit of most people's stomachs, especially if money is already tight. It isn't pleasant to think that the future of your family could depend on your ability to pay for a costly procedure that might not even work. Money is at the root of much marital tension to begin with—add the stresses of infertility to the mix, and the result is anything but peaceful.

As I think through all the things that can steal our joy during infertility, I keep coming back to one central theme: loss of control. This affects everyone to some extent, but it is especially true for overachievers and perfectionists (myself included) who have always been able to work, think, or talk themselves through any problem they've ever encountered. Unfortunately, infertility isn't like a complicated math problem or a difficult essay question. No amount of studying can make conception occur. No amount of persuasive talk can produce a positive pregnancy test. No amount of sweat or elbow grease can reverse a miscarriage. And for people who are used to being in control, such a predicament can be very disconcerting, if not downright scary.

This loss of control is often accompanied by an equally trying source of mental anguish—uncertainty about the future. This one hit close to home for me. After all, I'm the one who always reads the end of a novel first. This habit drives Randy crazy—he thinks it ruins the story. But I just like to know how things are going to end. With infertility, though, we can't turn to the last page in the book. The journey—no matter how long or how short—is littered with unknowns: "Will I *ever* be able to have kids?" "Are we going to run out of money before we run out of treatment options?" "How long should we try to conceive before we give up?" "What should we be doing now to prepare us for whatever's going to come next?" Infertility would be so much easier to deal with if we could just see how it was going to turn out. Or so it seems.

More Medical Issues

A lack of a clear diagnosis only makes the loss of control that infertility patients experience more painful. For many people, "Why can't I get pregnant?" is the question of the month—month after month. Sadly, the answer is often a mystery, even to doctors with years of specialized training.[2] It's easy to get discouraged when test after test fails to reveal any abnormalities. How do you correct a problem when you don't even know what the problem is?

Then there's the monthly emotional roller coaster. Who would have thought that trying to have a baby could turn a normally stable, rational, well-adjusted woman into a basket case? On the other hand, what else would you expect? In the early stages of treatment, you're careful to do everything right, from using store-bought ovulation predictor kits to lying on your back for an hour after intercourse. Nothing happens. Months later, a vaginal ultrasound reveals several good eggs, and the doctor says your husband's sperm count is perfect for the artificial insemination he's about to do. Still nothing. The higher you allow your hopes to rise, the worse you feel when your period comes—again. "Hope deferred makes a heart sick," Proverbs 13:12 says. Too much more of this, and you fear your heart condition will become terminal.

The mental and physical discomfort that accompanies visits to an infertility specialist can often be another cause of anxiety. It was for me and Randy. In fact, when I asked him to name the times during our infertility journey when he felt the least amount of peace, his answer was immediate: whenever we went to the clinic of the reproductive endocrinologist who performed my last two surgeries.

This particular clinic is affiliated with a university hospital. As such, it is very short on the comfort-providing touches you might find at a privately funded facility. Actually, there's nothing comforting about the place at all—from the stark linoleum floor and hard chairs in the waiting room to the cold blue walls in the examining rooms and the matter-of-fact bedside manner of the specialist.

It's not that he was incompetent or unpleasant. He was neither. But to say I dreaded going there is an understatement—I hated it. I hated the vaginal ultrasounds. I hated being treated like a number instead of a person. I hated the way procedures such as in vitro fertilization, the doctor's specialty, were promoted without the mention of any ethical concerns a patient might have about them. I even hated the hotel where we always stayed when we went to that particular clinic.

Yet another cause of uneasiness for couples facing infertility is the wide range of treatments that exists these days. Fifty years ago, couples who couldn't conceive naturally had two options: adopt or remain childless. Today, thanks to amazing advances in assisted reproductive technology, a whole menu of options is available, from potent drugs such as Clomid and Pergonal to high-tech procedures such as IVF, GIFT, ZIFT,* and others. But although these therapies and procedures provide hope in previously hopeless situations, they also can confront infertile couples with ethical dilemmas that they would never have had to deal with before.

Frozen embryos, multiple births, and "selective reduction" suddenly are much more than subjects in a reproductive endocrinology textbook—they are very real issues with very serious moral and ethical implications. What type of reproductive assistance is appropriate for a Christian to receive? How far is too far? What if your doctor, the one to whom you are turning for help in this deeply painful trial, recommends something, but you're not sure if it's right for you? What if he says it's your only chance, but you still can't decide? No wonder you have trouble sleeping at night.

You might think that, once you get away from the doctor's office, your turmoil would lessen a bit. That might be true if there were no other people in the world. But that's simply not the case. Everywhere you turn, you run into women who look like they're about three days away from going into labor. It's bad enough with strangers, but when the pregnant women are your friends or relatives, it's even worse. You can't help but look at them and wonder why *they* are getting what you so desperately want. And then there are all those other people who seem to think it's their life mission to give you advice or "encouragement" about your situation. No matter how many times you tell yourself they have no idea what you're going through, their comments still sting.

---

* IVF: in vitro fertilization; GIFT: gamete intrafallopian transfer; ZIFT: zygote intrafallopian transfer. See chapter 8 for more information.

Worse yet, these comments can make you question your most deeply held beliefs and convictions. Which brings up my final—and most significant—reason why peace is often hard to come by during infertility. Your questions about why you can't get pregnant might be directed to your doctor at first, but inevitably they turn upward. And when those questions—those agonizing prayers—just seem to bounce off the ceiling, everything you've been taught about God all your life is suddenly in jeopardy. Is it true? Is it real? Will it sustain you when your dreams begin to crumble around you?

That depends on what you've been taught—and on what you believe.

TWO

A Solid Starting Point

◦≈◦

*L*ong before Randy and I began thinking about having a child, we met a couple who had been trying to get pregnant for several years. Until we met these people, I had never personally known anyone who was dealing with infertility. When I was growing up, I occasionally heard about people—usually women from church—who couldn't have children. But the only thing I really remember about these ladies is that they seemed to cry an awful lot.

With our friends, however, it was different. Their infertility had caused serious problems in their relationship, to the point where they had even separated for a time. I felt bad for them because I could see that their unfulfilled longing for a baby was a source of intense pain. But I didn't really understand why not being able to have a child was such a big deal. I just didn't comprehend why they were so distraught about it.

My logical mind had it all figured out. *God is the only one who can create life,* I reasoned. *So if I were in their shoes, I would take comfort in knowing that, if He wanted me to be pregnant, I most certainly would become pregnant—and if I didn't become pregnant, it was because He had something else in mind for me.*

Now, looking back through a lens that has been scratched and chipped by personal experience, I'm amused that I even attempted to figure out their situation. I had no idea what infertility is like, no clue about the pain it entails, no notion of the theological struggle it triggers. My theory was rooted in truth. But had I expressed it, it would have fallen on deaf ears because I lacked one vital ingredient: empathy.

Fortunately, I had the good sense not to share my analysis with our friends. They went on to have several children, while I—well, you know what happened to me. I still lack many things, but empathy for people dealing with infertility is no longer one of them. And yet, though I now have an entire personal résumé of infertility experience, my basic belief about God's role in the whole thing really hasn't changed.

It doesn't look and feel quite the same, of course. Nothing does after having been stretched, pulled, yanked, and tested by the forces of uncertainty, physical suffering, and disappointment. During the last few years, my belief has been transformed from a one-dimensional, intellectual understanding to a deep, heartfelt conviction. Yes—God is in control of everything, including my infertility, and His plan for my life, whatever it entails, is good because *He* is good.

I can say that with confidence now—nearly a year-and-a-half after our last official attempt to get pregnant—because I'm starting to catch glimpses of what that plan might be. But like anyone who has faced a personal crisis of any magnitude, I had to wrestle with a number of difficult questions before I arrived at a place where I truly understood and believed it.

For infertility patients, especially those who are people of faith, the most difficult questions are often not related to medical concerns, as complicated as those may be. Instead, they strike at the core of who we are and what we believe about God: *Have I done something to deserve or cause this? Does God even care that I can't get pregnant? If He does care, why doesn't He do something about it?*

As I ponder my own bouts with such questions, I am convinced that Randy and I were able to have peace in the midst of our infertility largely because of our view of God and our understanding of how He relates to us as His children. And I'm just as convinced that there's a key reason many people do *not* have peace during infertility. It's because their view of God and His role in their lives is severely out of focus.

Because I believe this so strongly, I had determined that any book I might write about infertility had to include at least one chapter about God. I also knew that such chapters might be difficult to write because the people reading them would likely come from a wide variety of denominations and religious traditions. Some of you may have no spiritual background at all. Others may hold advanced degrees in various kinds of religious study. It's also possible that you may have begun your infertility journey with a firm set of beliefs, but have since become disillusioned because what you believed and what you're experiencing don't match up.

With that in mind, I want to share what I believe about God and explain how those beliefs provide the foundation for a healthy spiritual perspective on infertility. My thoughts are based on my own study of Scripture, what I have learned from trusted pastors, authors, and spiritual mentors over the years, and what I have witnessed in my own life and the lives of people around me. This chapter and the next one are simply a starting point, a framework upon which you can build a solid understanding of biblical truth about God's character and why He allows the type of suffering that accompanies infertility.

It's possible that what you're about to read might make you feel worse for a time. But if you let it simmer in your mind for a few days, weeks, or possibly even months (as I did), I hope it will eventually bring you the same measure of comfort and freedom that it has brought to me.

Seeing God As He Is

When I read personal stories about the emotional and spiritual aspects of infertility, I am always saddened by the amount of potentially avoidable confusion and pain in them. Jesus told His followers, "You will know the truth, and the truth will set you free" (John 8:32). Given all the untruths and partial truths about God, faith, sickness, and suffering that are tossed about in religious circles today, it's no wonder that freedom is the last thing that many infertility patients ever feel.

Ours is a performance-based society. We're conditioned to believe that, if we work hard—at school, at work, and even at home—we'll be rewarded for our efforts. It's a good system if the reward we're seeking is a good report card or a paycheck. But it doesn't translate so well when it's applied—as it so often is—to a person's relationship with God. We might get the basics down—that our salvation is a gift of grace from God, that we can do nothing to earn it, and that we certainly don't deserve it. But beyond that, we often fall into a trap. We think that, if we do what's right after we accept Christ, God will *always* show His approval by giving us good health and showering us with material blessings. And everyone knows that God's biggest, most important blessings have chubby cheeks, tiny fingers, and baby-soft skin.

This and other such beliefs might sound good on paper, especially when they're accompanied by carefully chosen Bible verses that seem to support them. But what happens when reality sets in? What if you are doing your best to honor God with your life and you just can't get pregnant, even though you desperately want a child? Does that mean that God is punishing you? That He no longer loves you? That He doesn't even care? That He does care but is unable to help because some sort of spiritual warfare is getting in the way? That He's not really in control after all?

Our understanding of who God is and how He works leads us to form certain expectations about how He is going to work in *our* lives. Sometimes that understanding is based on faulty or incomplete theology. Then we are set up for disillusionment when our expectations aren't met. As James Dobson writes in *When God Doesn't Make Sense*, "There is no greater distress in human experience than to build one's entire way of life on a certain theological understanding, and then have it collapse at a time of unusual stress and pain. A person in this situation faces the crisis that rattle[s] his foundation."[1]

The only way to avoid this kind of distress is to learn to "think theologically," as Charles Swindoll calls it. When we think theologically, we force ourselves to look outward and upward, to actively search for God's truth in the midst of all the spiritual distortions and misguided philosophies—and personal uncertainty—that swirl around and in us.

This practice is in stark contrast to what I tended to do in my early struggles with infertility, which was to focus solely on my pain, constantly wondering when God was going to show up and answer my prayers for a baby. Fortunately,

> God offers a better way to live—one that requires faith, as it lifts us above the drag and grind of our immediate little world, opens new dimensions of thought, and introduces a perspective without human limitations. In order to enter this better way, we must train ourselves to think theologically. Once we've made the switch, our focus turns away from ourselves, removing us from a self-centered realm of existence and opening the door of our minds to a God-centered frame of reference, where all things begin and end with Him.[2]

Thinking theologically doesn't come naturally—it takes self-discipline and perseverance. But the results—peace in the midst of pain and sadness, comfort in the absence of answers, confidence in the middle of uncertainty—are definitely worth it.

So where do we start? How do we go about formulating (or bolstering or refining) a foundation that will hold firm through the earthquakes of infertility? As far as I'm concerned, there's only one way to begin—by searching the Scriptures to find out the truth about God. Our source is reliable and trustworthy. Psalm 119 assures us that the Bible will show us the way—"Your word is a lamp to my feet and a light for my path" (verse 105)—and protect us on our journey—"Great peace have they who love your law, and nothing can make them stumble" (verse 165). That should give us confidence as we delve into our search.

God Is Close to the Brokenhearted

Throughout the Bible, God is described as our heavenly Father (Isaiah 9:6; Matthew 6:9; Romans 8:15). For those of us who are fortunate enough to have wonderful earthly fathers, this description brings with it a positive set of thoughts. I have no trouble thinking of God as a loving, personal being who cares for me and has my best interests at heart because that is exactly how my own father is. However, for people whose fathers are abusive, neglectful, harsh, aloof, or absent, the picture is entirely different. For them, the word "father" doesn't invoke feelings of warmth and security. Rather, it brings pain, hurt, sadness, and anger.

Our image of God is almost always connected in some way to our image of our earthly father. This helps to explain why so many people have great difficulty trusting God or understanding that He loves them unconditionally. The good news is that, even if family dysfunction or hurtful relationships are hampering your image of God, He *does* love you unconditionally. As the apostle

Paul says, nothing you do can remove His love from you. And nothing that happens around you can sever it either.

> *Who shall separate us from the love of Christ? Shall trouble or hardship or persecution or famine or naked-ness or danger or sword? As it is written: "For your sake we face death all day long; we are considered as sheep to be slaughtered." No, in all these things we are more than conquerors through him who loved us. For I am convinced that neither death nor life, neither angels nor demons, neither the present nor the future, nor any powers, neither height nor depth, nor any-thing else in all creation, will be able to separate us from the love of God that is in Christ Jesus our Lord (Romans 8:35-38).*

Those are powerful words. I remember how much comfort they brought me when, a few days after the tragedies of September 11, 2001, I heard President George W. Bush quote some of them during a prayer service in Washington, D.C. Happily, they don't apply just during times of national calamity. They also hold true during personal crises.

God doesn't love us from afar. He is intimately acquainted with every aspect of our lives, from our physical characteristics (according to Luke 12:7, He knows the precise number of hairs each of us have on our heads, which is truly mind-boggling for someone with hair as thick as mine) to our innermost thoughts and desires. If you're not sure about this, listen to David's words:

> *O LORD, you have searched me and you know me.*
> *You know when I sit and when I rise; you perceive my*
> *thoughts from afar.*
> *You discern my going out and my lying down; you are*
> *familiar with all my ways.*

Before a word is on my tongue you know it completely,
*　　O LORD.*
You hem me in—behind and before; you have laid your
*　　hand upon me.*
Such knowledge is too wonderful for me, too lofty for
*　　me to attain.*
Where can I go from your Spirit? Where can I flee from
*　　your presence?*
If I go up to the heavens, you are there; if I make my
*　　bed in the depths, you are there.*
If I rise on the wings of the dawn, if I settle on the far
*　　side of the sea,*
even there your hand will guide me, your right hand will
*　　hold me fast.*
If I say, "Surely the darkness will hide me and the light
*　　become night around me,"*
even the darkness will not be dark to you; the night will
*　　shine like the day, for darkness is as light to you.*
For you created my inmost being; you knit me together
*　　in my mother's womb.*
I praise you because I am fearfully and wonderfully
*　　made; your works are wonderful, I know that full*
*　　well.*
My frame was not hidden from you when I was made in
*　　the secret place.*
When I was woven together in the depths of the earth,
*　　your eyes saw my unformed body.*
All the days ordained for me were written in your book
*　　before one of them came to be.*
*　　　　　　　　　　　　　　　　—Psalm 139:1-16*

Because of the severity of my endometriosis, I get tripped up when I read the last few verses in this passage. How can someone with my set of health problems be considered "wonderfully made"? And yet, in God's eyes, I am. When He put me together in my mother's womb, He knew exactly what He was doing. Although I sometimes feel damaged and broken, He made no mistakes when He created me. He didn't forget a part or fail to finish a section. He made me just the way He wanted me.

And He made you just the way He wanted you.

God Will Not Forget Us

Because our heavenly Father loves us so much, He loves to give us good gifts (Matthew 7:9-11). But just like a kind earthly father, He sometimes withholds those gifts—those things we want so badly—because He has our best interests at heart. He knows what will be best for us (*and* perhaps give us the most joy) in the long run.

That's not to say He turns His back on our disappointment and sorrow, however. Even when things seem to be falling in around us or situations are not turning out the way we had hoped, God's love and care surround us. He is "close to the brokenhearted and saves those who are crushed in spirit" (Psalm 34:18). He promises to strengthen us, help us, and uphold us with His "righteous right hand" (Isaiah 41:10). He is forever faithful (2 Timothy 2:13), He is good (Psalm 136:1), and He never changes (James 1:17). As a result, we can rest in the assurance that He will never, ever forget us. One of my favorite passages in the entire Bible confirms this awesome thought: "Can a mother forget the baby at her breast and have no compassion on the child she has borne? Though she may forget, I will not forget you! *See, I have engraved you on the palms of my hands; your walls are ever before me*" (Isaiah 49:15-16).

But what happens when the burden of infertility gets to be almost more than you can bear? After three years of wildly irregular cycles, or six unsuccessful artificial insemination attempts, or three miscarriages, or—in my case—two major abdominal surgeries within eight months, it's easy to start thinking that maybe God has confused you with someone else. Maybe He actually *has* given you more than you can stand. But that is simply not true. No matter what the trial, no matter how hard it gets, His grace *is* sufficient for you, because His power *is* made perfect in your weakness (2 Corinthians 12:9). He knows how much pain you can bear. And although it's usually a lot more than you think, He will not allow it to crush you without providing some means of escape. He might not rescue you the way you expect Him to, but He *will* rescue you.

In the meantime, in the thick of the battle—when you feel you can't take another step (or face another period or doctor visit)— your heavenly Father stands waiting, arms wide open, to soothe your aching heart. "Come to me, all you who are weary and burdened, and I will give you rest," He whispers to your sorrowing spirit. "Take my yoke upon you and learn from me, for I am gentle and humble in heart, and you will find rest for your souls. For my yoke is easy and my burden is light" (Matthew 11:28-30).

Rest for my soul—now that was something I often longed for as I started to realize my desire for a child wasn't going to be fulfilled as easily as I had hoped. That rest came eventually, but not until I began to truly understand how other, less comfortable aspects of God's character were intimately involved with my infertility.

God Is in Control

You see, everything I've just written assures me of God's care and eases my anxiety about my worth and value. But it also brings up a whole new set of questions. If God loves me so much, why is He not answering my prayers for a child? Why is He letting me hurt so much?

These questions would pose quite a problem if God's character were limited to what I call His "loving-father attributes." His character certainly includes all of those things, but it encompasses much, much more. Now, if we were still focused on ourselves and our problems, this is where we might start to get frustrated, confused, and perhaps even angry. But we're trying to think theologically—upward and outward, remember? So let's continue our search of the Scriptures so we can get a more complete picture of God's character (as complete as our finite, mortal minds can grasp, that is).

When I was in elementary school, one of my Sunday school teachers taught a lesson that made a huge impression on my young mind. He introduced us kids to some pretty lofty principles about God—namely, that He is "omnipresent," "omniscient," and "omnipotent." To this day, I remember what those words mean: that God is everywhere at once (omnipresent), all-knowing (omniscient), and all-powerful (omnipotent). Said differently, God is present everywhere, He knows everything, and He is in control of everything.

That, in a nutshell, describes God's sovereignty, a biblical concept that sounds somewhat intimidating but is vitally important to this entire conversation. The fact that God is sovereign means that nothing happens in the world and in my life that does not first filter through His hands. He is in charge, even when a disease such as endometriosis destroys the fertility of an unsuspecting victim like me. He's also in charge when a baby is born dead, when a fatal illness strikes a young mother of four, when a car accident puts a vibrant teenage athlete in a wheelchair, when an unfaithful spouse refuses to repent, and when terrorists crash planes into tall buildings. He doesn't necessarily *cause* these things to happen—many are a direct result of the evil that pervades our fallen world. But not one of them occurs without His permission.

Remember Job, the Old Testament hero who suffered such great loss and yet refused to forsake his faith? Before Satan took away Job's business, family, and health, he had to ask God for permission. God gave it, but He also set certain boundaries that Satan was forbidden to cross (Job 1:12; 2:6). Satan was allowed to wreak havoc on Job's life for a time, but God was in complete control throughout the process. Job himself acknowledged this near the end of his testing: "I know that you can do all things," he told God. "No plan of yours can be thwarted" (Job 42:2).

God sees what we can't see. He knows what we don't know. He sees the big picture while we only know what's going on in our little world. As we deal with the day-to-day struggles of infertility, for example, He already knows the outcome. He knows when it will end, how it will end, and what will happen next. And He's in charge of the whole process, from start to finish.

Let me personalize this a bit. When I was getting ready for my second surgery, God already knew that it wasn't going to work and that in another eight months, I would have to do it all over again. He could have done something to make the surgery be successful the first time, but He didn't, perhaps because He had some greater purpose in mind.

How can someone with my set of health problems be considered "wonderfully made"? And yet, in God's eyes, I am.

This brings to mind Joseph, another Old Testament hero who was able to recognize that God's purposes had been fulfilled through his suffering. Joseph's brothers had sold him into slavery when he was a teenager. Years later, Joseph became the second most powerful man in Egypt. As such, he was responsible for preparing the country for an upcoming famine and for managing the distribution of stored food during the famine. He was reunited with his brothers when they came to Egypt in search of grain. Naturally, they were afraid he would seek revenge on them for what they had done to him so long ago. But their fears were unfounded. "You intended to harm me, but God intended it for good to accomplish what is now being done, the saving of many lives," Joseph told them (Genesis 50:20).

This story is a great example of God's amazing ability to "make silk purses out of sows' ears," as the saying goes. The apostle Paul restates this thought in the form of a promise—the promise that Randy and I clung to through our experience: "We know that in all things God works for the good of those who love him, who have been called according to his purpose" (Romans 8:28).

"All things" means just that. Everything. No exceptions. No exclusions.

But what exactly does that look like in everyday life?

THREE

His Ways Are Not Our Ways

If you're anything like me, you might find the idea that God's sovereignty encompasses "all things" a bit hard to grasp. Perhaps Charles Swindoll's description will help you put your hands around this amazing concept:

> His plan includes all promotions and demotions. His plan can mean both adversity and prosperity, tragedy and calamity, ecstasy and joy. It envelops illness as much as health, perilous times as much as comfort, safety, prosperity, and ease. His plan is at work when we cannot imagine why, because it is so unpleasant, as much as when the reason is clear and pleasant. His sovereignty, though it is inscrutable, has dominion over all handicaps, all heartaches, all helpless moments. It is at work through all disappointments, broken dreams, and lingering difficulties. And even when we cannot fully fathom why, He knows. Even when we cannot explain the reasons, He understands. And when we cannot see the end, He is there, nodding, "Yes, that is My plan."[1]

All the while, we're sitting here scratching our heads, wondering what in the world is going on. Our human minds simply cannot comprehend God's character, His behavior, or His activity in our lives (or seeming lack thereof). Try as we might, we just can't do it.

This really shouldn't come as a big surprise, however. The author of Ecclesiastes makes it very clear: "As you do not know the path of the wind, or how the body is formed in a mother's womb, so you cannot understand the work of God, the Maker of all things" (Ecclesiastes 11:5). And God Himself spells it out in big block letters for us: "'My thoughts are not your thoughts, neither are your ways my ways,' declares the LORD. 'As the heavens are higher than the earth, so are my ways higher than your ways and my thoughts than your thoughts'" (Isaiah 55:8-9).

In the New Testament, here's what Paul has to say about it: "Oh, the depth of the riches of the wisdom and knowledge of God! How unsearchable his judgments, and his paths beyond tracing out! 'Who has known the mind of the Lord? Or who has been his counselor?'" (Romans 11:33-34).

The answer, of course, is absolutely no one.

"Our God is in heaven; he does whatever pleases him" (Psalm 115:3). He answers to nobody. Nothing takes Him by surprise or catches Him unaware. He's not some Santa Claus in the sky, checking His records to see if we've been naughty or nice. He's not pacing the floor in the throne room, racking His brain to figure out how in the world He's going to make us get pregnant.

Nor is He obligated to give us biological children. Although we sometimes act like it, we have no right—constitutional, scriptural, or otherwise—to reproduce our genetic material. If God wanted us to conceive, however, it would happen in a millisecond. We're talking about the God who *spoke* the world into existence here. Although He often chooses to use us to accomplish His work, He doesn't *need* us for anything. He is the potter—and we are merely the clay (Isaiah 64:8). As such, *He* chooses the molds and uses whatever techniques He deems necessary to fashion us into the types of vessels He wants us to become.

His Plans, Not Ours

Let's go back to Job for a minute. A righteous man, Job could not figure out why he was being made to suffer so greatly. For 35 chapters, he vacillates between listening to his friends offer their flawed explanations and begging God to show up and explain what's going on. God shows up eventually, but He offers no answers. He simply fires a long series of questions at Job that very effectively put him in his place (Job 38–41). As author Frederick Buechner writes, "God doesn't explain. He explodes. He asks Job who he thinks he is anyway. He says that to try to explain the kinds of things Job wants explained would be like trying to explain Einstein to a little-neck clam."[2]

God understands our need to know why we're suffering—He made us, after all. He also understands our desire to know in advance how the story is going to end. Sometimes He gives us a glimpse of the reasons and perhaps even a clue about the end result. But most of the time, He simply asks us to trust Him. He asks us to believe that He knows how the story ends—that no matter what happens, He *will* work it out for our ultimate good.

This can be a difficult task, especially for those of us who would prefer to have our lives all organized and planned out for the next 20 years. We can get so caught up in mapping out our goals and our personal timetables that we forget that God might have something totally different in mind for us—something unexpected, and perhaps even unwelcome.

In the midst of all our planning, it's easy to forget that God simply doesn't think like we do. When Randy and I were trying to get pregnant, I often found myself thinking, *Okay, God, this would be the perfect time for me to get pregnant. The doctor just said that my chances of conceiving naturally are slim to none, and it sure would be awesome if You would step up to the plate and perform a miracle.*

It seemed like a good plan to me. In fact, if I were God, that's exactly what I would have done. But I'm not God and, as it turns out, He had something else in mind for me.

This reminds me of a passage of Scripture that I first came across during my senior year of high school or shortly thereafter. You're probably familiar with it: "'I know the plans I have for you,' declares the LORD, 'plans to prosper you and not to harm you, plans to give you hope and a future'" (Jeremiah 29:11).

God understands our need to know why we're suffering—He made us, after all.

In this passage, God is speaking specifically to the people from Judah who had been exiled to Babylon. But based on what we've learned about God and His character, we can infer that if God knew the plans He had for the Jewish captives, then He also knows the plans He has for us.

That's an extremely comforting thought, especially for recent graduates, people who are in the midst of great trials, and those who are on the brink of exciting change in their lives. But we have to be careful what we do with it. The verse says that God knows the plans He has for us—but I suspect that in our minds, we often revise it to say, "God knows the plans we have for *ourselves* (and of course He's going to work them all out so we can live happily ever after)."

That's simply not how it works. God's not a divine venture capitalist who sits at a big conference table in heaven accepting or rejecting life plans we submit to Him. The hopeful future we envision may look nothing like the future God has in mind for us. We imagine a life of happiness, ease, and relatively few problems, while God's plan might entail just the opposite. To us, prosperity and hope mean one thing—to God, they may look very different. That's because we see things through earthly, temporal eyes, while God views life from an eternal perspective.

You might look at your life today and think that not being able to have children is the worst thing that could happen to you. But God sees your life as it will be in five, ten, and fifteen years. Perhaps He knows that the joy, peace, and growth that you will experience in the future will come only as a result of your inability to get pregnant. And perhaps that's why His plans for you—"plans to prosper you and not to harm you, plans to give you a hope and future"—include infertility, at least for now.

Only He knows.

Which brings me back to that same old nagging question: Why?

Why is this happening to me? If God is so powerful, why doesn't He do something about this? Why, why, why?

Making Sense out of Suffering

It's not wrong to ask such questions. David, Job, and other Old Testament writers—men who walked closely with God— asked them all the time. As we've just discussed, the answers are usually elusive, if not downright incomprehensible to us as finite humans. But we can draw a few general conclusions about suffering from Scripture that might help make it easier to deal with the unanswered questions.

Let's start off by tackling the issue of whether infertility is a punishment. When Randy was a boy, he sincerely believed that he wasn't going to be able to have biological children, but would instead have to adopt. This was going to be God's way of punishing him for being mean to his younger brother, who is adopted. Now why in the world would an otherwise normal boy think this way?

The answer is simple. Randy grew up believing that God was a stern judge who was just waiting for His followers to mess up so He could "thump" them. Under this system, God's approval was gained by good works, and His disapproval was stirred by "bad works" (such as the typical boy's "mistreatment" of his little brother).

Randy no longer views adoption as a punishment. Rather, he now looks at it as a wonderful way to expand our family. But many people who have trouble getting pregnant continually struggle with whether they have infertility problems because God is angry with them for some reason. The Bible does include a few examples of women whose infertility or loss of a newborn child was a direct result of a specific sin. For instance, after Saul's daughter Michal criticized her husband, King David, for dancing in front of the ark of the Lord, the Bible records that she "had no children to the day of her death" (2 Samuel 6:23). Most of the time, however, we are not given any indication that barren women in Scripture were childless because God was punishing them. In fact, Elizabeth and Zechariah, the barren couple who miraculously conceived John the Baptist in their old age, were described as being "upright in the sight of God" (Luke 1:6).

I'm not suggesting that infertility is never a *consequence* of past sins and poor moral choices. We know that abortions and certain sexually transmitted diseases can damage the reproductive organs enough to prevent conception from occurring.[3] And though God lovingly forgives our sins, we still must live with the repercussions. In most cases, however, the causes of infertility—"anatomy, hormone function, sperm motility and quality, and hereditary factors—involve elements outside of the patients' control."[4]

You can never go wrong when you come to God during a trial and ask Him to reveal any hidden sins or areas in which you need to repent. Make it a habit to pray as David prayed: "Search me, O God, and know my heart; test me and know my anxious thoughts. See if there is any offensive way in me, and lead me in the way everlasting" (Psalm 139:23-24). But don't allow Satan—or anyone else, for that matter—to trick you into thinking that your infertility is a sign of God's disapproval or punishment. It's not.

Sometimes, in fact, God allows suffering so that He can demonstrate His power in a person's life. For example, Jesus once met a man who was born blind. His disciples assumed that the man's blindness was caused by his sin or his parents' sin. But they were wrong. "Neither this man nor his parents sinned," Jesus said before He healed the man, "but this happened so that the work of God might be displayed in his life" (John 9:3).

Such miracles still occur today, but they're certainly not guaranteed. No matter how godly or holy we are, we cannot escape the problems that pervade our fallen world. God may choose to heal our infertility, but He may not.

When Randy was a child, he learned a song that went something like this: "No sins, no sickness, no diseases, no infirmities, shall come against this house when Jesus is Lord." Sadly—or happily, for our eternal good—God made no such promise. In fact, He promised just the opposite. "In this world you *will have trouble*," He told His disciples (John 16:33). Thankfully, He softened the edges of that blunt reality in His very next breath: "But take heart! I have overcome the world."

So what's the message here? Are we just to accept suffering as a fact of life, something we have to endure until we die and go to heaven? Not exactly. Suffering is a fact of life, but it is also a great tool for spiritual growth. It's not necessarily the tool I'd choose for myself, but it is extremely effective. God knows what's best for us, remember? He sees us as we are, but He also knows what we can become. He knows exactly what it's going to take to mold us into His image, and His refining plan often includes some kind of suffering.

You might look at your infertility merely as an obstacle to overcome or a giant to conquer so you can move on to something better. To God, however, it might be the very tool He uses to draw you closer to Him. The apostle James recognized this truth: "Consider it pure joy, my brothers, whenever you face trials of many kinds, because you know that the testing of your faith develops perseverance," he wrote. "Perseverance must finish its work so that you may be mature and complete, not lacking anything" (James 1:2-4).

God Is Good

We might be able to come up with a few good theories about why God allows suffering and why He might have allowed our infertility. In the end, however, we just don't know for sure. We "see through a glass, darkly," and our vision will remain blurred until we see Jesus face to face (1 Corinthians 13:12, KJV). As much as we might learn about God and His work in our lives, there's infinitely more we will never be able to understand. As Charles Swindoll explains,

> There are some times when those who know the most simply must back off with hands behind their back and say, "It's beyond me." I don't know why God closes some doors and opens others....I don't know how evil can be used for good. And I don't know how the interplay between the two in some way glorifies God. But I know ultimately it does and it will, because God will be all in all. I don't have to explain it.[5]

On his 2001 recording, *Declaration*, Steven Curtis Chapman included a song that beautifully captures the essence of what I have learned about God and suffering as a result of my inability to conceive. The chorus goes like this:

> "God is God and I am not. I can only see a part of the picture He's painting. God is God and I am man, so I'll never understand it all. For only God is God."[6]

It's short. It's to the point. But most importantly, it's true.

In *When Empty Arms Become a Heavy Burden*, Sandra Glahn and William Cutrer, M.D., assert that the discussion about why God allows us to suffer boils down to two questions: "Is God good?" and "Will I trust Him?"[7] I didn't really understand how significant God's goodness was to all of this until I read a series of historical novels by Michael Phillips called "The Secrets of Heathersleigh Hall." A particular passage made such an impression on me that I just had to include it in this chapter. I think you'll see why when you read it.

Here's the scenario. A woman named Hope had served for a time as a missionary in New Zealand. She and her husband were enjoying their ministry and expecting their first child when a leader in their village turned on them, killing her husband and burning their home. The shock of it sent her into labor, but the baby didn't survive. This tragedy forced Hope to totally rethink her faith. "How can I believe in God's goodness after what has happened?" she asked herself over and over again.

She sank into deep despair. Then one day, after she had returned home to London, a chance opportunity to help a lost little boy find his mother made her realize that, despite her doubts and self-absorption, she was still capable of kindness and goodness. Upon recognizing that the goodness within her had come from God, she came to the conclusion that God truly was good. No, His goodness wasn't meant to take away the world's suffering, but it did provide a refuge in the middle of it. This realization transformed the way she looked at life.

> "What I came to accept was simply this…that *God is good*."
>
> A long silence followed.
>
> "Only that and nothing more," Sister Hope added, "—*God is good*.
>
> "It does not mean that things in my life will always be good…but that *God is good*. It does not

mean that my life will be an easy one…but that God is good. It does not mean that my prayers will always be answered in the way I would like…but that God is good. It does not mean that tragedy may not visit me…but that God is good. It does not mean that there will not always be suffering in the world…but that God is good. It does not mean that there will not be times when I am so overcome by sadness at memories in my life that I must go outside and find a place to be alone and just cry for an hour…but that God is good. It does not mean that there will not continue to be many who will deny his very existence because of the pain and seeming unfairness of life they see all around them…but that God is good. It does not mean that there will not always be many questions for which we have no answers…but that *God is good.*

"God's goodness is the larger truth over the whole, the largest truth overspreading all of life— over cruelty, over suffering, over tragedy, over doubts, over despair, over broken relationships, over sin itself. Why God's goodness doesn't eliminate such things, I don't know. Perhaps we shall ask him one day. For some reason our tiny human minds cannot comprehend, God has allowed suffering in his universe. I don't know why. You and I might have done it differently. But then we are not God, so it is impossible for us to see all the way into the depths of the matter. We therefore cannot perceive the many ways in which the very suffering we rail against may in fact contribute to the overall eternal benefit and growth of God's universe and its created beings.

"We cannot see to the bottom of such things. So we foolish creatures look at the world's suffering and say God must not exist, or if he does he must not care, or must be a cruel God. Yet I suspect that when we are one day able to see all the way into it, we will see that Goodness and Love lie at the root even of all the suffering that was ever borne by this fallen humanity of which we are part. The devil is presently having his brief illusion of triumph, but God's goodness will reign in the end."

She paused, then added, "In short, the circumstances of life do not always seem to be good, but God *himself* is always good. Thus, though there may not always be happiness, there *is* always hope. That must be the basis for our faith—not that God gives us a happy life."[8]

The first time I read that passage, it took my breath away. A few years later, it still hasn't lost its impact.

"Is God good?" Yes, absolutely. After reading Sister Hope's words, I hope you're convinced.

"Will I trust Him?" Ouch. The second of the two questions is a little tougher to answer.

Trusting Our Good God

It's hard enough to trust someone you can see, hear, and touch. With God, we have to trust someone who is invisible and silent, at least when it comes to our normal way of communicating. And yet, it is only when we put our trust in God that we can expect to experience true peace. Isaiah 26:3-4 (another one of my favorite Scripture passages) makes this clear: "You will keep in perfect peace him whose mind is steadfast, because he trusts in you. Trust in the LORD forever, for the LORD, the LORD, is the Rock eternal."

Trust is based on an informed choice. I choose to trust Randy based on what he tells me, what he does, and what I know about his character. I don't see everything he does because I'm not around him 24 hours a day. But I know he is an honest, honorable man who desires to please God with his life. Therefore, it's easy for me to trust that he will be faithful and good to me. If I were to hear that he had done something questionable, I would evaluate it based on whether such a deed was consistent with what I know is true about him. If it wasn't, I would seriously doubt whether what I had heard was true.

The same principle applies to my relationship with God. I choose to trust Him based upon what He says in His Word, what I know about His character, and what I see Him doing in the world around me. Sometimes events in my life or things people say plant seeds of doubt in my heart. At those points I return to what I know to be true about God: that He is faithful, that He does not lie, that He is just, that He loves me, that He is merciful, that He is sovereign, that He does not change. This knowledge bolsters my faith and reminds me that God is truly trustworthy—no matter what anyone tells me and no matter how bleak my circumstances might seem.

I realize that it can be hard to trust God if you have difficulty trusting people. But if you're struggling in your efforts to trust God, it doesn't mean that you're not a good Christian. It means that you're human. God knows the desires of your heart, and if you truly desire to trust Him, He'll show you how. Remember the man who wasn't quite sure whether God could heal his demon-possessed son? "I do believe," he told Jesus—"help me overcome my unbelief!" (Mark 9:24).

Jesus helped him, and He wants to help you, too. All you have to do is ask.

The Next Step

Whenever I think about what my infertility has taught me about God, His character, and His work in our lives, I'm always drawn back to the Old Testament book of Isaiah. The following section, taken from the fortieth chapter, inspires awe in my heart and comforts my spirit every time I read it. When you start to wonder whether God cares about you and your infertility—or whether He's really in control of the world and all its troubles— refer to these verses.

He tends his flock like a shepherd:
He gathers the lambs in his arms
and carries them close to his heart;
he gently leads those that have young.

Who has measured the waters in the hollows of his hand,
or with the breadth of his hand marked off the heavens?
Who has held the dust of the earth in a basket,
or weighed the mountains on the scales and the hills
in a balance?
Who has understood the mind of the LORD,
or instructed him as his counselor?
Whom did the LORD *consult to enlighten him,*
and who taught him the right way?
Who was it that taught him knowledge
or showed him the path of understanding?

...Do you not know?
Have you not heard?
Has it not been told you from the beginning?
Have you not understood since the earth was founded?
He sits enthroned above the circle of the earth,
and its people are like grasshoppers.
He stretches out the heavens like a canopy,
and spreads them out like a tent to live in.
He brings princes to naught
and reduces the rulers of this world to nothing.
No sooner are they planted,
no sooner are they sown,

no sooner do they take root in the ground,
than he blows on them and they wither,
and a whirlwind sweeps them away like chaff.

"To whom will you compare me?
Or who is my equal?" says the Holy One.
Lift your eyes and look to the heavens:
Who created all these?
He who brings out the starry host one by one,
and calls them each by name.
Because of his great power and mighty strength,
not one of them is missing.

Why do you say, O Jacob,
and complain, O Israel,
"My way is hidden from the LORD;
my cause is disregarded by my God?"
Do you not know?
Have you not heard?
The LORD is the everlasting God,
the Creator of the ends of the earth.
He will not grow tired or weary,
and his understanding no one can fathom.
He gives strength to the weary
and increases the power of the weak.
Even youths grow tired and weary,
and young men stumble and fall;
but those who hope in the LORD
will renew their strength.
They will soar on wings like eagles;
they will run and not grow weary,
they will walk and not be faint.

—Isaiah 40:11-14,21-31

The truth about God in this passage gives us a solid support to which we can cling during the tumultuous ride of infertility. And that brings me back to my pre-infertility analysis of how a person should cope if she were to have trouble getting pregnant. Although I had no idea what I was talking about back then, I've discovered that what was then just theory actually works in real life. During the years when Randy and I were trying to conceive, I derived great comfort from my deep conviction that, if my sovereign God wanted me to be pregnant, all the endometriosis in the world couldn't prevent it from happening. Ironically, I was also comforted by knowing that, if God had other plans for me, the best assisted reproductive technology man had to offer couldn't make me pregnant.

God alone is the one who opens and closes the womb. And though I still have to wrestle with the unanswered questions, the disappointments, and the pain, I'm secure in the knowledge that He loves me and that He is in control.

True Relaxation

After hearing that you're having trouble getting pregnant, has anyone ever advised you to "just relax"? If I've heard that bit of "wisdom" once, I've heard it a thousand times. And every time I hear it, it sounds even more ridiculous. No amount of relaxing will melt away the scar tissue and adhesions that prevent me from conceiving. It just won't happen.

That said, there is one type of relaxation that is beneficial to couples who are trying to conceive. I like to call it "relaxing in God's sovereignty." Ponder that phrase for a moment. You may have never thought to put the two words together. After all, "relaxation" brings to mind peace, tranquility, and solace, while "sovereignty" triggers thoughts of power, control, grandeur, and majesty. Yet, what better place can we be than relaxing in the loving arms of the omnipresent, omniscient, omnipotent Maker of the universe?

When I'm relaxing in God's sovereignty, I'm resting in the assurance that God knows what He's doing even if it doesn't make any sense to me. Relaxing in God's sovereignty frees me from worry. It relieves my anxiety. It brings me peace. And it gives me the freedom to say, "I don't know why this is happening to me—and that's okay."

FOUR

How to Pray

⚜

*I*t was the beginning of a new Sunday-school year at church. The education department had restructured classes for married adults into "Seasons of Life" groups and added a class just for people like us—childless couples who had been married five years or more. We were visiting with friends during the pre-lesson fellowship time, when a casual acquaintance who was aware that we were trying to get pregnant walked by.

"So what class are you guys going to?" he asked.

"We're obviously not going over there," Randy said, gesturing to where the "Parents of Preschoolers" group was gathering. "So we're going to try 'Just the Two of Us.'"

"Well," this jovial father of two said cheerfully, "we'll just have to pray harder."

With that, he turned and headed down the hall.

Somewhat used to off-the-cuff and ill-informed infertility advice by this time, Randy and I just looked at each other and rolled our eyes. But our friend's comment still touched a nerve. I'm sure he didn't mean it this way, but his words implied that, if we just persevered in prayer a while longer, if we just conjured up a little more faith, or if we groaned and cried a bit more while we implored God for a baby, then we most certainly would achieve the result we wanted.

I wasn't particularly upset by his comment, but I've never forgotten it. It sticks in my mind as one of the more insensitive nuggets of "wisdom" we've received over the years. But it also highlights one of the most bewildering questions associated with infertility: how to pray.

Biblical Models

What *is* the best way to pray for a baby? Is there a formula to follow, a key verse to meditate on, or a biblical example to emulate? Even if we wanted to, there's no way we could ever read all the books about prayer that are available these days, so how in the world are we supposed to come up with a good "infertility prayer strategy"?

Randy and I have a friend who, when she was struggling with infertility, asked just about everyone she knew to pray that she would get pregnant. She knew that James 5:16 says that "the effectual fervent prayer of a righteous man availeth much" (KJV), and she figured that the more people she asked, the better her chances that at least one of the people praying for her would fit into the "righteous" category.

But what about those of us who are a bit more private about our infertility journeys? What if we're not comfortable with the cover-all-the-bases method my friend used? I certainly don't fault anyone who prays for a baby with every breath and recruits others to do the same. If that's how you are moved to respond to your situation, more power to you. I have to tell you, though, that Randy and I took a different approach. And—to borrow a phrase from Robert Frost—that has made all the difference, not only in our response to our infertility, but also in the rest of our lives.

I suppose we could have focused on the examples of people like Hannah, Jabez, Job, or King David. We certainly wouldn't have been alone, especially if we had made Jabez our model. And yet, when we began trying to get pregnant, knowing full well that such an endeavor would probably be difficult, we chose to look to a different example in the Bible.

We took our cue from Jesus and the way He prayed in the garden of Gethsemane just a few hours before He was betrayed and arrested. Deeply sorrowful about the trial He was about to endure, Jesus asked His three closest disciples to keep watch while He prayed. He went a little ways away, fell with His face to the ground, and uttered one of the most profound prayers ever recorded: "Father, if you are willing, take this cup from me; yet not my will, but yours be done" (Luke 22:42).

What exactly was Jesus asking God for in that prayer? I'm no theologian, but it seems to me that He was contemplating the horrible pain His body was about to go through. He was pondering the excruciating agony of being separated from His heavenly Father. And in His humanity, He longed for another option. He knew He had come to earth to die on the cross, but as the hour of darkness loomed, He prayed for some kind of divinely approved release from that responsibility.

Knowing that Jesus was fully human, just as we are, it's easy to see why He asked God for another alternative—not once, not twice, but three times as He prayed in the garden. To me, the remarkable aspect of His prayer was the way it ended: "Not my will, but yours be done."

As a red-blooded human being, Jesus certainly preferred not to go through an agonizing death on the cross. And yet, even as He prayed for deliverance, He reaffirmed His submission to His Father's will. While His body screamed for another way, His soul and spirit were willing to accept the path He knew was before Him.

Christ's interaction with God the Father in Gethsemane is far more mysterious than I could ever hope to comprehend. The theological implications boggle my mind. In that hour, did Jesus—fully man and fully God as He was—really not want to die?

Is it possible that God could have said "yes" to Jesus and rolled out what we might think of as Plan B, much like He did with Abraham when he was about to sacrifice his only son, Isaac, on Mount Moriah (Genesis 22)? I don't know the answers to these questions. I only know how our elementary understanding of Christ's experience in the garden helped Randy and me pray for a baby.

How We Proceeded

Using Jesus' words as a guide, we regularly reminded God that we really wanted me to get pregnant. We made no bones about it. We knew that God had created us with an inborn desire to procreate, and we knew that our desire to have a baby was not wrong. So we let Him know how we felt, no holds barred. But every time we prayed, we also expressed to Him that what we wanted, more than anything else in the world, was His will for our lives. Yes, we really wanted a baby, but if He had something else in mind for us—well, we wanted His will to be done. In other words, if His plan for us didn't include a biological child, then we didn't want a biological child.

For me, that prayer started out more as an intellectual exercise than a true heartfelt desire. As you might guess, the prayer was difficult to pray. I really did want to get pregnant and have the chance to experience all the little events and feelings that go along with a pregnancy. For some reason, though, the thought that I might miss out on God's best if I insisted on my own way made me keep praying that way.

And as month after month passed without a pregnancy, an interesting thing began to happen. The more we prayed that prayer, the more it worked its way from my mind to my heart, until it truly did become my heart's desire. After a while, I really started to mean it. I can't explain how this happened—I just know that it did.

There were times, however, when I felt that praying this way signaled a lack of faith. After all, I had friends who were consistently storming the gates of heaven about their infertility or adamantly holding on to their belief that God was going to allow them to get pregnant. Meanwhile, I sometimes felt as if I were hanging on to an escape clause, giving both God and myself a way out in case my prayers for a baby weren't answered the way I

Yes, we really wanted a baby, but if He had something else in mind for us—well, we wanted His will to be done.

---

wanted. I knew, beyond a shadow of a doubt, that He *could* make me pregnant, no matter what the doctors said. But I didn't know whether He *would*. And at times I felt as if praying this way was my own little way of protecting myself and keeping my expectations in check.

I'm not quick to blame every problem or trial on the work of Satan. But I am quite certain that these doubts I occasionally had did not originate with God. So whenever such thoughts popped up, I quickly squelched them by reminding myself of the peace I was experiencing. I wasn't worrying. This, as I will explain in a later chapter, was a miracle in and of itself! I wasn't fretting. I wasn't agonizing over what was going to happen to me in the future (again, another drastic change from the way things used to be in my life).

It's not that I didn't experience all the usual bouts of grief and disappointment that go along with infertility. I did. But through it all, I knew that I was praying for God's will to be done. Based on everything we talked about in the previous two chapters, I knew He was hearing my prayers. So the only logical conclusion I could come to was, no matter what happened, God's will *was* being done. Even if I wasn't getting pregnant.

This might sound odd, but I derived a tremendous amount of comfort from that thought. That comfort, coupled with the peace I felt, deflated my doubts about whether I was praying the right way. I had the peace that transcends understanding, and that was all I needed.

Roadblocks

I realize that what I'm advocating is not easy to do. I also want to stress that Randy and I didn't begin praying this way because we were some kind of superspiritual saints. More than anything else, we prayed this way because we didn't know what else to do, and because we couldn't stand the thought of missing out on God's calling in our lives.

That said, I know there are significant roadblocks to this type of prayer. Not the least of these is the deep desire that most infertile couples have to get pregnant and give birth to a healthy baby. One verse keeps coming to mind: "Delight yourself in the LORD and he will give you the desires of your heart" (Psalm 37:4). Sometimes we mistakenly believe that this verse promises us that, if we love God, He will give us everything we want. But even if we understand the true meaning of this verse intellectually (that when we delight in the Lord, His desires for our lives gradually become our desires), the incorrect belief can still distract us and ambush our emotions—especially when people around us seem to get the desires of their hearts quite easily.

So what do we do when our intense desire for a child gets in the way of our ability to pray that God's will be done in our lives, no matter what that will might be? What I'm about to suggest might sound a bit harsh, especially because the Bible emphasizes what blessings children are and what an honor it is to have them. For now, however, we have to set that aside and focus on the immediate situation. If you are experiencing infertility, you have to at least acknowledge that having a biological child is one blessing that you might not get to enjoy, at least for now. You can allow your deep desire for a child to make you depressed and bitter. But perhaps a better solution would be to ask God to lessen your desire, or perhaps take it away entirely.

Does this show a lack of faith? No—I think it is a healthy way of dealing with reality. You're not halting your prayers for a baby—you're simply asking God to make your infertility journey a bit easier.

Does asking God to change the desires of your heart actually work? I believe it does. It happened to me, and it happened to my friend Carmen Jones. In her case, however, the desire she had to give up was perhaps even more significant than the desire for a baby.

I met Carmen when I was writing my first book, Women, Faith, and Work. Though her story doesn't involve the inability to have a child, it is definitely relevant. When Carmen was 20, she was involved in an automobile accident that left her paralyzed from the waist down. For many months following this terrible event, Carmen truly believed that God was going to heal her and allow her to walk again. It took her a couple of years to work through the denial and begin to accept her new status as a paraplegic. How did that finally happen? Here's how she explained it to me: "I just began to ask God to change my desire from walking to fully living life: 'If I'm going to live this life, you've got to show me how I can live it.' And he began to change my heart so that walking wasn't such a big deal."[1]

More than 15 years later, Carmen can say, without a moment's hesitation, that the accident was the best thing that ever happened to her. It deepened her relationship with Jesus in ways she never could have imagined. It also led her to her current career as the owner of a small business that helps corporations market their goods and services to disabled people.

Carmen's story touched me deeply when I first heard it. But it wasn't until I was proofreading my book that I made the connection between her prayer about walking and what God had done for me in regard to my desires for a biological child. As I read her words, something finally clicked in my mind. We had prayed for God's will regarding our family. And I realized that He had, to paraphrase Carmen, changed my heart so that getting pregnant and giving birth to a child wasn't such a big deal. It was a wonderful realization, to put it mildly.

My point in telling you this story is simple: If your strong desire for a child is interfering with your ability to pray for God's will, consider asking God to soften that desire and make it more bearable. You might be surprised at what happens next.

There is another roadblock I want to mention. Considering it cuts straight to our innermost thoughts and motivations, leaving no ugly stone unturned. As you read the previous paragraphs, perhaps you found yourself stamping your foot and saying to yourself, *I don't even want to entertain the thought that, in order for God's will to be done in my life, I might have to release my dream of getting pregnant and having a baby. I just won't do it. I want a baby too much.*

If this describes you, your biggest problem is not infertility. It's a lack of submission to your heavenly Father.

I know that might sting. It's not exactly the easiest thing I've ever written, that's for sure. But it's the truth. It comes down to this: Do you want what you want, or do you want what God wants? Are you willing to give up your wants and desires, no matter how honorable and natural they might be, so that He can be free to rule sovereignly in your life? If you never get to that point, you will never experience true peace, no matter how many children you might end up having. Never.

Honest to God

I know this is a lot to dump on a person who is hurting. And yet, dealing with these core issues might be the only way you can work through your pain and experience the joy of relaxing in God's sovereignty.

So where do you stand? Maybe you're ready to start praying for God's will, regardless of whether or not that includes a baby. If so, go for it. Blessings await, I promise you.

On the other hand, maybe you'd really like to be able to pray that way, but you're not sure you can do it honestly. Perhaps you'd like to ask God to change your desires, but you're not sure you really want Him to. Or maybe you've just recognized the painful truth that you simply aren't willing to submit this area of your life to God—not right now, and perhaps not ever.

Whatever the case, there is hope. Once again, the answer lies in prayer. No matter what your situation, the first step is to tell God exactly how you feel. Tell Him that you want to pray for His will, but your will is getting in the way right now. Tell Him you want Him to change your desires, but you're afraid to let go of that dream. Tell Him you want to believe that He will hear and answer your prayers, but your faith is weak and you're growing tired. Tell Him that you know you have a submission problem, and you really don't want to do anything about it. Wherever you are, just begin the conversation.

Don't be afraid to express your honest emotions. It's better to tell God how you feel, even if it's extremely negative, than it is to keep it all bottled up. It's not like He doesn't already know how you feel, anyway. If you think it's somehow inappropriate to express anger, disappointment, or bitterness to God, think again. Time and time again, the writers of Scripture freely shared their feelings with their Maker. Job did it. Jeremiah did it. So did David, the very person the Bible describes as a man after God's own heart. "How long, O LORD? Will you forget me forever?" he asked. "How long will you hide your face from me? How long must I wrestle with my thoughts and every day have sorrow in my heart? How long will my enemy triumph over me?" (Psalm 13:1-2).

That certainly doesn't sound like someone who was afraid to voice his feelings to God, does it? He wasn't disrespectful, but he didn't shy away from saying what he thought. Follow David's example and don't hold back, even if you sense your anger might be verging on sin. Just tell Him about your emotions. He can handle it.

This reminds me of an experience one of my former college professors shared with me when I returned to campus years later to interview her for a newspaper article. Dr. Shirley Thomas grew up in a small town in Arkansas and married at the ripe old age of 16. Six years later, when she gave birth to her second son, she was shocked to discover he had Down's syndrome. This unexpected problem made her extremely angry—at God, and at everything else.

A preacher's wife with a decided flair for the dramatic, Dr. Thomas has always dealt with grief or anger by eventually "having a fit on God or somebody." She stayed true to form when her son was born. When he was a few months old, she put him in a little seat and took him out to a hillside, where she tried to pray.

> [I] just had a mad, screaming, cussing fit at God and explained to God that I could do a better job of running the universe than he could...The bitterness that was there just really poured out. I knew from reading the Bible [that] the scripture says that God will not put on you more than you can bear. And I told God that he had made a mistake, that I couldn't bear this."[2]

Dr. Thomas was numb for several months after this incident, but her "fit" allowed the healing process to begin. It can be the same with you, if you'll just open up and let God know how you're feeling. I repeat, He can handle it.

Hang On for the Blessing

The changes that will occur in your heart and life as you pray for God's will to be done probably will not be immediate. This can create quite a challenge for those of us who are used to living a fast-paced, results-oriented life. Our society is so geared toward instant gratification and instant success. We're accustomed to using pagers, cell phones, fax machines, and credit cards to get what we want when we want it. Such technology has its place, but when this kind of thinking spills over into our prayer life, the results aren't pretty. We want answers, and we want them now. If the answer we want doesn't come as quickly as we think it should, we often get frustrated and angry.

Just tell Him about your emotions. He can handle it.

As we discovered in the last chapter, however, God doesn't operate according to our schedule. His ways are simply not our ways. He doesn't have to give us monthly progress reports, and He certainly doesn't owe us an explanation every time He says "no" or "wait." So when it comes to your infertility prayer strategy, persistence is a key ingredient.

Don't give up. Remember Jacob, the Old Testament patriarch who had an all-night wrestling match with God? "When the man [God] saw that he could not overpower him [Jacob], he touched the socket of Jacob's hip so that his hip was wrenched as he wrestled with the man. Then the man said, 'Let me go, for it is daybreak.' But Jacob replied, *'I will not let you go until you bless me.'"* (Genesis 32:25-26).

As you pray through your infertility, take your cue from Jacob and hang on for the blessing. It might not come in the form you're expecting, but it will come. In the meantime, ask God to take away your worry and your fears. Ask Him to replace them with peace and contentment. Know that when you pray this way, you are praying according to God's will—after all, His Word says that "godliness with contentment is great gain" (1 Timothy 6:6).

There may be times during your infertility journey when you feel as if your prayers are bouncing off the ceiling. You might be diligent in asking God to increase your contentment and help you to trust Him more, but it seems as if you're not making any progress at all. What then? If you are really struggling with issues such as submission, contentment, or trust, you might want to think about doing something a bit more drastic. You might turn to the biblical practice of prayer and fasting—perhaps for a few meals, a few days, a week, or even longer—to help you achieve the spiritual breakthrough you so desire. I'm not suggesting some kind of quid pro quo fast where you give up food in exchange for a baby (although if God calls you to fast for healing from infertility, I certainly wouldn't discourage you from doing it). I'm talking about giving up food for a time in order to allow God to work on your heart. He can tear down strongholds of selfishness, discontentment, unbelief, lack of submission, or anything else that might be interfering with your ability to pray for His will to be done in your life.

I realize that prayer and fasting might be a foreign concept to you. It's not talked about much in the church today. It is entirely biblical, however, and it can be a source of great spiritual growth and blessing if you choose to do it. If you want to know more, see Appendix C for a resource that can help you begin.

Prayer Support

If your infertility journey drags on for any length of time at all, there will probably be times when you find you are too tired to pray. It's not that you've given up hope that God is listening—it's just that you've repeated yourself so often that you just can't handle doing it one more time. Maybe you've thoroughly thought over your situation and prayed about it from every conceivable angle until there's just nothing left to say. Or maybe you're so emotionally drained—perhaps from a procedure that didn't work or yet another month gone by without a pregnancy—that you just don't know what to say. You feel as if you need to keep praying about your infertility, but you just don't have the energy.

I often felt that way when we were praying for a baby. At times like that, two things gave me strength and hope. First, I clung to a promise in Romans 8:26-27:

> The Spirit helps us in our weakness. We do not know what we ought to pray for, *but the Spirit himself intercedes for us with groans that words cannot express.* And he who searches our hearts knows the mind of the Spirit, because the Spirit intercedes for the saints in accordance with God's will.

I derived great comfort in knowing that, when words failed me and when I was too weary to pray, the Holy Spirit was interceding on my behalf, lovingly reminding the Father of what my heart didn't know how to express.

The other thing that kept me going was the knowledge that friends and family members were faithfully upholding Randy and me in prayer. Because I knew our parents, siblings, and close friends were bringing our desire for a child to the throne of God regularly, I didn't have to feel bad if I went for a couple of days or a week without reminding Him that we wanted a baby.

Even as I write these words, I can imagine questions that might arise. *How can she expect God to answer her prayer when she doesn't even have enough strength to persevere? What kind of faith is that?* I asked myself the same things. But in the end, I had to trust that God knew my heart. He knew I wasn't being lazy and relying on other people to do what I should have been doing myself. One of our responsibilities as believers is to bear each other's burdens, and I am eternally grateful for the people in my life who bore my burden of prayer—at least about this issue—when I just couldn't do it.

A word of caution is in order: If you ask too many people to pray for you, you might find that you are constantly fielding questions about your "progress." This can become exhausting. I suggest that you find two or three close, trusted friends—people you know are true prayer warriors—and recruit them as prayer partners. If you want this to be completely effective, be specific about your prayer requests. Don't just ask them to pray you'll get pregnant. Ask them to pray the way you are praying—that God's will be done in your life, and that you will have the strength to accept it, whatever it might be. If you are struggling with a particular issue, whether it is contentment, or submission, or an upcoming procedure, ask them to pray about it. And don't forget to let them know when something good happens—as seemingly "minor" as an encouraging conversation with someone, or as "huge" as a positive pregnancy test.

The End Result

As you put the finishing touches on your infertility prayer strategy, don't forget these three steps: "Be joyful always; pray continually; give thanks always, for this is God's will for you in Christ Jesus" (1 Thessalonians 5:16-17). Obedience to this passage, coupled with a commitment to pray the way Jesus prayed in the garden, will change your heart and life in ways you might never have imagined. You will come to experience tremendous freedom—from worry, from anxiety, from fear, and from despair and disillusionment. And the best part about it is, this freedom won't affect just your infertility journey. It will spread to other parts of your world and transform the way you see life in general.

Trust me—the results are worth it. Even if they don't include a positive pregnancy test.

FIVE

God Sightings

❧

*N*o matter how theologically solid your infertility prayer strategy is or how committed you are to following it, there are bound to be times when you get discouraged because God doesn't seem to be answering your prayers for a baby.

You've probably heard the little adage about how His answer is often "no" or "wait." But when months or years go by without a dramatic answer to prayer, it's easy to lose heart. It's like taking a cross-country road trip and never stopping to spend the night in a hotel or to see one single tourist attraction along the way. You know your goal is to get from New York City to Los Angeles as quickly as possible, but by the time you reach Kansas City, you're so tired of driving that you don't think you can go another mile. Had you broken up the trek with an overnight visit with friends in Philadelphia or a short visit to the Arch in St. Louis, the excursion might have been bearable. But because you didn't plan for any fun stops, the trip seems as if it will never end.

The infertility journey is the same way. There are times when it seems as if God is oblivious to your prayers and you wonder if you will be asking Him for a baby until you die. Thankfully, however, you are not doomed to a life of constant discouragement. During those long periods of "silence," one of the ways you can keep from losing heart is by intentionally looking for what I like to call "God sightings." I'm not talking about seeing an image of Jesus in the clouds or finding the face of God on the side of a building. Rather, God sightings are those often-overlooked little events and moments that gently remind us that our heavenly Father still loves us and is still working. Even when it comes to our infertility.

My friend Joyce has a wonderful practice of pointing out "coincidences" that, in retrospect, don't seem quite so coincidental. A casual flip through a magazine leads to an exciting job opportunity. A chance meeting with a friend provides a bit of encouragement just when you need it the most. An unexpected day off during a very hectic month gives you a chance to get caught up on some important correspondence with your family. The magazine flip, the chance meeting, the day off—they might seem like coincidences, but they could all be considered God sightings, even if you don't recognize them as such at the time.

God sightings can happen in all areas of life. But it's especially crucial that you learn to notice—and remember—the ones that relate to your infertility journey. That's because, perhaps more than anything else, they serve as tremendous faith-builders. As you experience one God sighting after another, always making a point to record them in your mind or on paper, they combine to form a base to which you can return when your faith grows weak. They become part of your history, a chronology you go back to again and again as you reflect on what God has done for you.

That's what the children of Israel did throughout the Old Testament. When they came together as a group, their leaders would often trace their history—from God's covenant with Abraham, Isaac, and Jacob to the great deliverance from Egypt, from the giving of the Ten Commandments to the entrance into the promised land, and so forth. The purpose of these recitations was simple: They reminded the people—adults and children alike—that the God of the Hebrews was the one true God, the only One worthy of service and worship.

There is one big difference between their experience and ours. They and their ancestors actually *saw* God, or at least a bit of His glory. Abraham walked and talked with the Lord (Genesis 18). Moses saw the burning bush (Exodus 3). The children of Israel saw Moses' face glowing after he had been in God's presence on the mountain (Exodus 34:29-35). God typically doesn't reveal Himself like that anymore—rather, He communicates with us through His written Word, the Bible. But He still moves in ways we can detect, which is what God sightings are all about.

Heavenly Affirmation

Let me give you some examples so you'll know exactly what I mean.

I'll start with an early God sighting, one that happened before Randy and I got married. You might recall that my first surgery was done to remove a grapefruit-sized cyst from one of my ovaries. Several months before the surgery, I got sick with some kind of intestinal bug. When I went to the doctor, I was told my sickness was "going around" and would go away soon. It didn't. I returned to the doctor. Again, I was told the malady would go away. This time, however, I also was instructed to drink lots of milk (why, I don't know). My problems continued, so after a few weeks, the doctor finally decided to do some tests.

This is where the story gets interesting. A minor exam of my lower colon somehow indicated I was lactose-intolerant (which explained the continuation of my problems after I was told to drink more milk). And a significantly more uncomfortable procedure revealed I had some kind of mass protruding into my colon. That led to the sonogram that unveiled the cyst. In this case, the God sighting was the illness that prompted me to go to the doctor in the first place, plus the instruction to drink lots of milk, which led to more problems, which led to the tests.

Despite the severity of my endometriosis, I had never experienced any symptoms that I was aware of, and if it hadn't been for my bout with the intestinal bug, there's no telling when my condition would have been diagnosed. Looking back, it's clear to me that God was orchestrating events even then to bring about His ultimate plan in my life.

There are times when it seems as if God is oblivious to your prayers and you wonder if you will be asking Him for a baby until you die.

Let's scoot forward a few years to August 1997. I had just stopped taking birth control pills, and Randy and I were looking forward to starting a family. We also were looking for a new house. (We were in the process of selling our first home to our next-door neighbor.) We searched high and low for a house we liked that was in our price range and big enough for our future family, but we kept coming up short. Then we found a new neighborhood, the Lee Valley subdivision, in a small town on the outskirts of our city.

At the time, the real-estate agent helping the developer market Lee Valley was a grandmotherly lady named Cil. We liked her as much as we liked the subdivision, and we began to look at lots and possible floor plans for a new house in the neighborhood.

One Saturday, I was thinking about becoming a mother and feeling down because I didn't think I would be a very good one. I cried, and Randy prayed for me. That evening, we went to the subdivision to look at an existing home with Cil. Afterwards, she mentioned that the little boy who lived in the house had taken quite a shine to me.

"You're going to make a good mother," she said as we walked to our cars.

Talk about an affirming touch from God! It brings tears to my eyes even now, more than four years after we moved into our peaceful home in Lee Valley. The experience affirmed to me once again that God cares about our deepest needs, and that He delights in soothing our hearts and easing our fears.

Spiritual Healing

As a God of incredible grace, He's also kind enough to help us when the trouble we are having stems from our own sinful tendencies. In my case, that sinful tendency was my lifelong propensity to worry, especially about health issues. I had my diagnostic laparoscopy in mid-January 1999. As I explained in chapter one, the surgeon took one look at the condition of my internal organs and decided to refer me to a specialist. At the time, my biggest worry was that our health insurance wouldn't pay for my medical care because we were trying to get pregnant and the plan didn't cover infertility expenses.

I was also worried about whether the specialist my doctor wanted me to see was part of the network of healthcare providers approved by our insurance. This might seem like a small thing to fret about. But to me, it was a big deal. And you know what? When Randy called to see if the doctor was part of the network, he learned that the specialist had been added to the list the week before we called.

How gracious of God! Even as He saw me mired in worry and failing to trust Him, He was going ahead of us, taking care of the details that I was so obsessed with and opening doors for what needed to happen next.

Although it might seem somewhat insignificant in the grand scheme of things, this God sighting was huge for me. It was a key turning point in my battle with worry—something that was so much a part of me that my brothers and sisters had nicknamed me "Worry Busby" as a child. Though I had often prayed to overcome it, it practically consumed me at times. I worried about articles I was writing, things I might have forgotten to do, accidents or other tragedies that might happen to someone I loved—you name it, I had it covered.

As I began to pray for God's will to be done in my life as far as a baby was concerned, however, the seeds of transformation slowly began to germinate. Little by little, as I began to trust God for something over which I had absolutely no control, I began to worry less. And not just about things I couldn't control.

I didn't even realize this was happening until I was driving home from work one spring day, shortly after my first appointment with the specialist. I can't remember what I was thinking about, but it suddenly occurred to me that I had not had a worrisome thought for several weeks. You may not fully grasp the magnitude of that thought—but for me, it was a God sighting if there ever was one.

As I continued to drive, I realized that, although God had not elected to heal me from my endometriosis and infertility (at least not yet), He had, in effect, healed me from my worrying. Some people might dispute such an application of the word "healing," but in my opinion, that's exactly what happened. I was healed, mentally and spiritually. My husband can attest to this. If he had the chance, he would tell you what a stranglehold worry had on my life, and how different I am now. He would also tell you that he would much rather have no children and a wife who doesn't worry than two or three babies and an obsessive, constantly fretting wife (which is exactly what I would have been had God allowed me to get pregnant before my problem with worry was resolved).

This is not a prideful boast. I'd be the first to admit that my tendency to worry was something I was powerless to overcome. Rather, it is a humble and grateful acknowledgement of the fact that, even when my prayers for a baby seemed to be going unanswered, God was still focused on my life, lovingly defeating an enemy that had plagued me for so long. And as Eugene Peterson's paraphrase of Philippians 4:7 so beautifully states, "It's wonderful what happens when Christ displaces worry at the center of your life" (THE MESSAGE).

A little more than a year and two major surgeries later, I experienced another God sighting. This one happened on the day after Mother's Day. We had a postoperative appointment with the specialist, and while we were there, we asked him to outline for us our chances of conceiving with various procedures. I had done enough reading to know what he was going to say, but we wanted to hear him say it.

As we suspected, the news wasn't good. According to the doctor, I had a 0 to 1 percent chance of conceiving naturally, a 7 to 10 percent chance of conceiving through artificial insemination, and a 35 to 40 percent chance of getting pregnant via in vitro fertilization. For reasons I will explain later, we had already ruled out in vitro, so our pregnancy outlook was pretty bleak.

Such an announcement might have been totally devastating, especially since it came the day after Mother's Day. But even as the doctor was talking to us, my heart was filling with a peace I can't explain. I didn't get upset. I don't think I shed even a single tear. It wasn't denial that made me so calm—it was the assurance that God was in control.

Later that week, I got some very positive feedback at work that affirmed to me I was doing exactly what God wanted me to be doing at that time. The peace continued to flow. I was relaxing in God's sovereignty like never before, even as my chances of getting pregnant seemed to be fading into the distance.

Start Looking

By now, you should have a pretty good idea of what a God sighting is. Perhaps my anecdotes have triggered memories of times when you sensed God's presence and felt His loving embrace, even in the midst of sadness and disappointment. I hope so. It's also possible that, at this point, you might be unable to acknowledge anything besides a positive pregnancy test as a God sighting. If that's the case, don't give up. As you learn to pray for God's will to be done in your life, you will begin to feel His presence, and it will become easier to detect other God sightings as they occur.

Many of the things I describe in this chapter happened before I heard the term "God sighting." I knew the experiences were special when they happened—I just didn't have a clever-sounding name for them. Other things, such as the events leading to the discovery of my original cyst, were only recognizable as God sightings after the fact. That doesn't detract from their ultimate faith-building potential—it just shows that sometimes it takes a while for us to become aware of their significance. Most importantly, when I consider them individually and as a whole, I can't help but be amazed by the fact that this awesome God actually cares about me. And like the Israelites of old, I'm reminded that He alone is worthy of my worship and service.

Wherever you are in your infertility journey, make a concerted effort to notice God sightings as they happen. It's fun to watch them unfold, and it's exciting to look back and remember how God showed up when you least expected Him.

That's exactly how I feel when I think about the last two God sightings I want to share with you. One happened to me, the other to Randy. The interesting thing about these experiences is that they both happened during our first visit to the gynecologist who is now my doctor.

A Divine Embrace

I'll tell my story first. After the specialist explained our chances of conceiving, we decided to try artificial insemination once or twice. We left his office with a prescription for Clomid and instructions to call him as soon as an ovulation-indicator test revealed that I was about to ovulate. I took the fertility medication and followed the doctor's instructions about the timing of the ovulation tests. But I never got a positive result.

This was strange because I always ovulated around the same time every month. It was also extremely frustrating. Our doctor's office was in a city about three hours away, and every day I got up expecting that we'd have to make the trip there the next day, only to be disappointed when yet another test failed to give the result we needed. To make matters worse, the whole time I kept having doubts about whether this was what we were really supposed to be doing. I was so tired of surgeries, uncomfortable procedures, medical offices, hospitals, and waiting rooms.

By the end of the week, I had made up my mind. I was never going back to that specialist. I was done trying to have a baby.

Randy agreed with me about the doctor, but he wasn't quite ready to give up on conception. So we decided to see if we could find a good local doctor who might be able to do some minor infertility procedures for us. I discussed our needs with my friend Tina, who was a labor and delivery nurse at a local hospital at the time. We wanted a compassionate doctor, I told her, one who would listen to us, seriously consider our preferences, and not try to push anything on us that we didn't want to do.

Tina is one of those caring people whose very presence provides comfort to a hurting soul. She understood exactly what I was going through, and she recommended a doctor she had often worked with at the hospital. I made an appointment, but I didn't want to go. In fact, I was dreading it. I couldn't stand the thought of another pelvic exam or vaginal ultrasound.

The day of the appointment came. Randy and I met at the doctor's office. My stomach churned, and the muscles in my neck and shoulders were tight. Although the waiting room was warm and cozy—more like the lobby of a luxurious hotel than a women's clinic—I really didn't want to be there.

I was sitting at a table filling out paperwork when the outside door opened and in walked Tina. She had gotten a last-minute appointment for a regular checkup with this same doctor (one of the privileges of being a nurse, I guess), and her time slot just happened to be a few minutes before ours. I'll never forget how I felt when I saw her. It was as if a warm breeze came in the door with her and blew away every last trace of the anxiety and fear I was feeling. The minute I saw her, I knew everything was going to be okay. I can't really explain it. I just knew her presence there—for a last-minute appointment that could have happened anytime— was an answer to my prayers. Some might call it a coincidence— I call it a God sighting.

As I sat in my car afterward and pondered what had happened, I was overcome with emotion at the thought that God had allowed Tina to be there at the doctor's office exactly when I needed her comforting presence and reassuring words. I don't think I've ever felt more loved and cared for by God than I did that morning.

Randy's Turn

I didn't know it at the time, but that visit to the doctor was very meaningful for Randy also. Before I explain why, some background is in order. As I mentioned in the first chapter, Randy was at my side before and after every surgery, even before we got married. He accompanied me to every doctor's appointment, procedure, and test when we were trying to get pregnant. He held my hand and told me to breathe when the doctors were poking and prodding me with uncomfortable instruments. He tried to distract me when I was getting blood drawn or IV tubes inserted into my arm. He sat with me in waiting rooms, helped me get dressed after every exam, and prayed for me when I needed strength. If it hadn't been for him, there is no way in the world I would have been able to go through any of this.

As a man who takes his role as my provider and protector very seriously, it was very difficult for Randy to just sit there while all this was happening to me. But the experiences at the doctors' offices pale in comparison to what he went through during and after my surgeries. The most recent one was the most difficult. The night before, I had to drink a gallon of what someone in the pharmaceutical profession had the gall to call "Go-Lightly." This awful drink is designed to totally clean out the colon, and it does its job well. The only problem is that it is extremely tough to drink this stuff at the prescribed rate of one cupful every ten minutes, especially after it begins to work.

The only thing worse than doing this at home is doing it in a hotel room. That's what I had to do. About two-thirds of the way through this ordeal, I couldn't take it anymore. I threw up all over the bathroom and all over Randy. Although I made a big mess, he never complained. He just wrapped me up in blankets, put me on the bed, and cleaned up the bathroom.

The next day, he sat in the waiting room at the hospital, first with me as we waited (and waited and waited) for me to be called to surgery, and then by himself during the nearly four-hour procedure. Having never been in that situation, I can't even imagine what it must be like. I just know that waiting for the doctor to come out with his report must be incredibly nerve-racking and scary. But for Randy, the worst was yet to come.

My surgery was on a Tuesday, and I didn't leave the hospital until Sunday. That whole time, he sat by my side on a hard window seat, reading a book, speaking softly to me when I woke up, watching as nurses and aides occasionally tried to squeeze drops of blood out of me, and trying to cope with all the smells coming from my very stinky roommates. At one point, I had no less than six tubes coming out of me—one for oxygen, one sending liquid to the epidural in my back, and another draining fluid from my abdomen, plus two IVs and a catheter. I must have been a pitiful sight.

Perhaps the lowest point for Randy came the day after my surgery, when I decided I wanted to get up and walk around. I had done this fairly easily with each of my other surgeries. I didn't expect any problems this time. But I didn't realize that because I had lost a significant amount of blood during surgery—not enough for a transfusion, but almost—getting out of bed so soon was going to be quite a challenge.

I made it to the edge of the bed a time or two. Each time, though, I decided to lie back down. On one of these attempts I discovered that my catheter tube wasn't draining right because it had gotten tangled up somehow. Randy told the nurse about it, and she decided I needed to stand up so she could untangle the tube. I managed to get up, but soon felt weak again. The aide was busy fixing the tube and didn't want me to lie down just yet. I then started to slump, as if I were going to faint. But instead of helping me down, the aide kept trying to prop me up.

At this point, Randy decided to intervene. Telling the aide I needed to sit didn't spur her into action, so he physically moved her out of the way and started to lay me down on the bed. (At this, she got mad and left the room.) By this time I was totally white and very clammy. To make matters worse, when I began slumping over, I also started convulsing as if I were having a seizure. Understandably, this scared Randy to death.

"Why is she doing that?" he asked the other aide who was standing by watching the whole episode.

"I don't know!" she exclaimed.

At this point, he was getting panicky. "Why is she doing that?" he demanded again, practically yelling at her this time.

"I don't know," she protested again as she rushed out of the room, never to return.

Even before he had begun questioning the aide, Randy had correctly assumed that I was struggling because there wasn't enough blood reaching my brain. He swiftly lowered the head of my bed, and I stopped convulsing. Eventually, his heart slowed down enough to allow him to resume his regular post on the hard window seat next to my bed.

Wherever you are in your infertility journey, make a concerted effort to notice God sightings as they happen.

The whole episode had lasted only about 15 seconds. But for Randy, it was one of the single worst experiences of our whole infertility journey. It confirmed his feeling that he didn't want me to have to go through endometriosis surgery every year for an unforeseen number of years. If I ever had to have surgery on my reproductive system again, he wanted it to be the last time.

I've told you all this to set the stage for our visit with the new gynecologist. As I said before, the atmosphere at the clinic was cozy and inviting, as was the little office where we met with the doctor. We liked him immediately. He was warm and personable, but more importantly, it was clear that he had carefully studied my medical records and knew everything that had happened to me in recent months.

"I've had a chance to review your chart, and it's a long one," he said after greeting us. "I'm not going to do any tests on you today because it looks to me like you've been poked and prodded quite enough."

You've been poked and prodded quite enough. Those seven words were music to Randy's ears. Finally, here was a doctor with years of medical training who openly acknowledged what my kind, compassionate husband had been feeling for some time—that I had been through enough. Randy was so happy to have his own concern validated that he almost hugged the man.

For Randy, it was a God sighting of mammoth proportions.

After discussing our options with the doctor, we went on to do three intrauterine inseminations. When the last one failed, we tearfully closed one chapter of our lives and moved on to the next one. We were finished trying to get pregnant. We would now start thinking seriously about adoption.

We weren't about to forget what had happened to us, however. As we started the adoption process, we were encouraged by the God sightings we had witnessed—on that hot July day at the doctor's office, as well as during the previous months and years. Little by little, they had made our faith stronger, giving us a solid foundation that we could stand on as we waited for our family to grow in another way.

SIX

Avoiding the Comparison Trap

❦

*R*ecalling these special times when we sensed God's presence and saw His hand at work in our lives can provide a wonderful break from the more troubling realities of infertility. Unfortunately, such breaks are usually temporary. Wherever we go, we're bombarded with reminders of what we don't have—pregnancy-test commercials on television, baby-shower invitations, crying infants in shopping malls, child-dedication ceremonies at church, and so on.

Perhaps the most difficult reminders of all, however, are encounters with pregnant women. It doesn't matter if the expectant mother is a dear friend, a sister, a co-worker, or a stranger at Wal-Mart, there's just something about seeing a growing tummy on someone else that can trigger a rush of tears, a bout of melancholy, or a round of depression that can linger for hours, if not days.

I know the Bible tells us to rejoice with those who rejoice, and I suppose that includes being happy for all the expectant parents we know. But as anyone dealing with infertility can attest, that can be a daunting—if not nearly impossible—assignment.

The intensity of our reactions to other people's pregnancies can be surprising, even alarming. Who would have thought comments such as "We weren't even trying" or "We really don't need another kid" could spark such feelings of anger or bitterness. If the pregnant person happens to be an unmarried teenager or someone who can't seem to handle the children she already has, the emotional response is even stronger.

For people struggling with infertility, such scenarios tend to release a flood of indignant questions: "Why does *she* get another kid when she can't even manage the ones she has?" "Don't you know she doesn't even *want* any more children?" "Does she *really* believe that having another child will keep her husband from leaving?" "What right does a promiscuous teenage girl have to become a mom?"

No matter where these questions start, however, they all eventually lead back to the same basic, nagging one: *Why her and not me?*

This type of struggle doesn't begin with an infertility diagnosis, of course. We start learning the pattern at an early age, from the first time we experience something that our little minds perceive as unfair. "How come Suzy gets to stay up later than me?" "Why does Sam get to go to the party and not me?" "Why does Jennifer get to be the team captain instead of me?"

As we get older, the scenarios change. Instead of unwelcome bedtimes, our displeasure stems from disparities we encounter at work or unfavorable comparisons with other people's lifestyles or possessions. But regardless of whether we're dealing with an older sibling, a neighbor, a co-worker, or a stranger on the street, the root problem remains the same: our natural tendency to focus on other people and the ease with which they seem to get what we want.

Such comparisons rarely produce positive results. But when it comes to infertility, they can be downright harmful. Few things can steal our joy and rob our peace faster than our very human inclination to compare ourselves and our family situations to other people and their family situations. Without getting over-dramatic, I believe it's one of the most effective tools Satan uses to discourage us and make us angry and resentful—toward God and toward other people—as we attempt to get pregnant.

Encounters with pregnant strangers—at ballgames, restaurants, concerts, or wherever—aren't as conducive to comparisons, because unless you live in a very small town, you'll probably never see these women again. But when the expectant mothers are friends or close relatives, the dynamics change entirely. You want to be happy for your loved ones. You don't want your sad circumstances to detract from their joy. At the same time, you can hardly bear to be around them because their protruding bellies constantly force you to acknowledge your own inability to conceive.

As bad as it sounds, it's even worse when the expectant mothers are former infertility patients. Whoever coined the phrase "misery loves company" knew what he was talking about. It's a lot easier to commiserate with someone who shares your suffering than it is to rejoice when that person's suffering ends and yours doesn't.

So what's the answer to this difficult comparison problem? You could always move to a remote mountain cabin. You'd probably never see a pregnant woman there, but even if it were possible to move, you'd still have to deal with birth announcements and pregnancy news via e-mail, the telephone, and the U.S. Postal Service. Staying holed up at home for the duration of your infertility journey is another option. Shopping for groceries over the Internet would get old very quickly, though, and missing months of church and work wouldn't be good for your spiritual or financial well-being. There's really only one practical alternative: learning to handle other people's pregnancies in an emotionally healthy, spiritually mature way.

A Lesson from Narnia

In case you're wondering, I didn't sit down one day and decide that I really needed to get a handle on my emotions toward pregnant women. In fact, I can't remember exactly when Randy and I stumbled upon the concept I am about to share with you. I just know that it has literally transformed the way we look at other people's pregnancies. It's given us a way to handle all the fertility "unfairness" we see around us without going crazy.

A few years ago, we began reading C.S. Lewis's Chronicles of Narnia out loud together, usually before we went to sleep at night or in the car on long road trips. I had read the series twice before, once as a child and once as an adult. At first, Randy probably wouldn't have admitted that he was actually reading the whimsical children's books, but it wasn't long before he was as hooked as I was.

Our "aha" experience came in the car, en route to some vacation destination. We were reading *The Horse and His Boy*, which traces the adventures of a little orphan named Shasta, an aristocratic runaway named Aravis, and two talking horses as they all attempt to travel to Narnia. We had come to the part in the book where Shasta finally meets Aslan, the lion that rules Narnia (and the character who serves as the Christ figure in Lewis's allegory). Shasta encounters Aslan on a foggy mountain path, but because he can't see him, he doesn't know what he is. He's afraid Aslan is a ghost. But when he feels the lion's warm breath on his hand and face, he relaxes a bit and begins to share his litany of sorrows.

He tells how he had been orphaned at a young age and raised by a stern fisherman. He tells how he had then escaped. He tells how he and his companions had been pursued by lions at least twice and how one lion had actually gotten to Aravis and wounded her. He tells about all the other dangers they have faced on their journey to Narnia. And he also tells about their trek through the desert and how terribly hungry and thirsty and exhausted he is.

"I do not call you unfortunate," said the Large Voice.

"Don't you think it was bad luck to meet so many lions?" said Shasta.

"There was only one lion," said the Voice.

"What on earth do you mean? I've just told you there were at least two the first night, and—"

"There was only one: but he was swift of foot."

"How do you know?"

"I was the lion." And as Shasta gaped with open mouth and said nothing, the Voice continued. "I was the lion who forced you to join with Aravis. I was the cat who comforted you among the houses of the dead. I was the lion who drove the jackals from you while you slept. I was the lion who gave the Horses new strength of fear for the last mile so that you should reach King Lune in time. And I was the lion you do not remember who pushed the boat in which you lay, a child near death, so that it came to shore where a man sat, wakeful at midnight, to receive you."

"Then it was you who wounded Aravis?"

"It was I."

"But what for?"

"Child," said the Voice, "I am telling you your own story, not hers. I tell no one any story but his own."[1]

This entire passage paints a beautiful picture of how God protects us and lovingly guides our paths, even when we don't realize it. But it was the last two sentences that grabbed our attention and wouldn't let it go.

I am telling you your own story, not hers. I tell no one any story but his own.

An Amazing Discovery

When I read those 18 words to Randy, it was as if a huge light bulb turned on in our minds. The message was clear: The things that happen in the lives of other people—including their pregnancies, no matter how undeserved or unwanted they may be—are part of "their story." It is neither our responsibility nor our business to know why God allows them to happen.

Talk about a revelation! It was as if God were saying, "You know how you're always comparing yourselves to other people and asking me why they're the ones getting pregnant when you're the ones doing everything right? Well, here's your answer. It's none of your concern! What happens to them has nothing to do with your life—it's *their* story and you don't need to worry about it!"

You might think I'm reading too much into this passage, but there's actually a biblical precedent for this idea. It's found at the end of the Gospel of John, during one of Christ's postresurrection appearances. After welcoming a repentant Peter back into His inner circle, Jesus proceeded to tell the humbled disciple the kind of death he was going to endure.

Intrigued by this glimpse into his future, Peter then wanted to know how the apostle John was going to die. But that bit of information was off limits. "If I want him to remain alive until I return, *what is that to you?*" Jesus said to Peter. "You must follow me" (John 21:22).

If we apply this principle to our infertility, here's what we might hear Jesus saying: "If I want your co-worker to have three babies in three years, what is that to you? You just focus on what I want *you* to do." "If I allow a woman from your infertility support group to get pregnant, what is that to you? You just take care of yourself, and let me handle everyone else." "If I let your best friend conceive unexpectedly, what is that to you? Your job is to obey and trust me. That's it."

It takes a lot of discipline to do this. You basically have to mentally separate yourself from what's going on in other people's lives and recognize that what is happening to them has nothing to do with you. The fact that your friend is pregnant and you aren't does *not* mean that she has God's blessing on her life and you don't. It simply means that God's plan for her right now includes a baby, and His plan for you right now does not.

Neither plan is better or more spiritual. They're different, to be sure, but that's just how life is. Although we can control some aspects of our lives, other areas are totally out of our hands. Had I been given the opportunity, I might have chosen the "have three kids by the time I'm 30" option, or I might have selected the "work until I'm 28 and then stay home with my newborn twins" alternative. But although other people are able to control their family planning, God didn't leave that choice up to me. His design for my life is a custom plan.

Close to Home

You might not think the "that's their story" mindset would make all that much difference when it comes to dealing with other people's pregnancies, but for Randy and me, it has made all the difference in the world. It was especially helpful when we heard that my younger sister, Esther, had gotten pregnant three weeks after her wedding. The timing of this totally unexpected announcement was terrible—at least as far as our infertility was concerned. At the time, we had been trying to get pregnant for nearly two years, and we were quickly nearing the end of the six-month window of opportunity that my second surgery had supposedly opened for us.

The news that Esther was pregnant could have been devastating to us. After all, we were the ones who had been trying so hard to conceive, while she and her husband Steve weren't even planning to start adding to their family for at least a year. And yet, remembering that she was living out her story and we were living out ours really helped us deal with all the conflicting emotions we felt. We knew that she and Steve would learn things from this experience that they might not learn any other way, just as we have learned (and continue to learn) lessons through our infertility that we probably wouldn't have learned any other way. God had one growth plan for them, and another for us. As long as we kept that in mind, we could be happy and excited for them.

Comparisons rarely produce positive results. But when it comes to infertility, they can be downright harmful.

It's also helpful to remember that just because other people get what we want so easily, it doesn't necessarily mean that their lives are perfect. Esther had all kinds of dreams and plans for her first year of marriage. However, those dreams and plans didn't include giving birth before her first anniversary. Although giving up her notion of the ideal first year of marriage might not have been as traumatic for her as giving up the dream of having a biological child was for me, it was still difficult for her. Her pregnancy involved the loss of dreams, just as my infertility involved the loss of dreams.

The truth is, we simply don't see other people's lives through their eyes—we only see them from the outside. It's easy to look at a woman with several children and say she has it made. But if we investigated a little further, we might discover that her marriage is foundering, her family is struggling financially, or one of her children has a special need that requires round-the-clock care. Sure, she may have the children that we so desperately want. But she might also have a lot of other challenges that we don't have to handle.

This is yet another reason why we need to avoid the comparison trap at all costs. There's always more to any given situation than meets the eye, and when we compare ourselves to someone else without having all the facts, we're only hurting ourselves.

Again, thinking like this is much easier said than done. But if it's the only way we can keep from becoming (or remaining) bitter, jealous, resentful, or depressed, we just have to buck up and do it.

Thanks to God's grace and the lesson we learned from *The Horse and His Boy,* we made it through Esther's pregnancy without any major emotional upheavals. These days, we can't imagine our family without little Warren, who is by far one of the most delightful tykes I've ever met. And we're also looking forward to the arrival of his little sister, Emma—yet another surprise who is bound to steal our hearts just as Warren did.

As I think back over the last few years, I'm amazed at the impact the "that's their story" concept has had on our response to all kinds of situations, not just ones dealing with other people's pregnancies. When something horrible happens to someone we love, and through our tears we can't help but ask God for an explanation, the answer is always the same: *I am telling you your story, not hers.* When immoral people around us prosper and we wonder why, the refrain repeats itself: *I tell no one any story but his own.* When someone else gets what we want—whether it's a new job, a promotion, an honor, or a baby—and we demand to know what's going on, the message is loud and clear: *What is that to you? You must follow me.*

Such answers might make us bristle at first. However, when we make a commitment to stop comparing ourselves to other people, our contentment level goes way up and our ability to rejoice with those who rejoice improves dramatically.

Continuing Education

Before I end this chapter, I need to make one more very important point. As wonderful as the "that's their story" approach is, it's not something you learn overnight. Nor is it one of those one-time courses that never has to be repeated. You might think you're doing really well coping with your infertility—and then all of a sudden, you're confronted with a situation that makes all the old negative feelings come rushing back.

I learned this the hard way several months ago. Not surprisingly, my emotional earthquake happened after a week that was full of opportunities for me to rejoice with other people. On Monday, I found out that my older sister Ruth was pregnant for the third time (after two miscarriages). The next day, Randy and I took dinner to some friends who had just had a baby. On Friday, I heard that a couple who'd had difficulty conceiving their first baby were expecting their second child, less than a year after the first one had been born. Finally, on Sunday, I discovered that some friends who had long given up their hopes for a baby had become pregnant unexpectedly. "Our miracle baby," they called him.

Each bit of news was joyous, each celebration delightful. Randy and I were smitten by our friends' new baby girl. We were both thrilled and anxious for my sister and her husband. And we were amazed that our friends who had accepted their infertility and gotten on with their lives were now preparing to become parents.

Under normal circumstances, none of these events would have fazed me. After all, I too had accepted my infertility and was looking forward to building my family through adoption. But when all this news came in one week—during a time of the month when my emotional stability was at its shakiest—it was too much for me to handle. Monday morning found me sitting on the couch in our living room, crying my eyes out and wondering why

I had to be the one who had to wait so long to become a mother because I couldn't have children the normal way. It might sound kind of odd, considering everything else we had been through, but I don't know if I've ever felt lower at any other time during our infertility journey than I did at that moment. I was simply overwhelmed.

My response was perfectly normal and understandable. But even as I cried, I knew I couldn't dwell on my sadness too long. I had to move on. I had to remind myself that, as much as I wanted to know why God was letting my friends and sisters experience this joy while I had to wait, it was really none of my business. Yet again, I was reminded that they are living out their stories and I am living out mine. And my primary job, as the main character in my story, is to focus on Jesus, not on anyone else.

It's a lesson we all have to learn time and time again. But it's worth repeating, because it goes such a long way toward helping us find and maintain true peace as we navigate the twists and turns of infertility.

SEVEN

Thick Skin, Soft Heart

*W*e've come up with a game plan for how to deal with other people's pregnancies. Now let's move on to what might be an even more frustrating aspect of infertility: all the medical advice, bits of biblical wisdom, and fertility folklore that people seem to feel compelled to share with you when you're having trouble conceiving.

I suspect that most, if not all, of you can recall at least one conversation in which a friend, family member, casual acquaintance, or total stranger asked you a question or made a remark about your efforts to get pregnant that left you annoyed, hurt, angry, or even completely dumbfounded. Many of you could produce a whole list of such episodes and be able to recount each incident in vivid detail. It's not that you *want* to remember these comments. It's just that they're often so insensitive or ignorant that you simply can't help it.

When Randy and I were trying to get pregnant, these irritating conversations often had to do with other people's experiences with endometriosis. It seemed as if everyone who learned of my condition had a sister, aunt, cousin, friend, or daughter-in-law who had suffered from endometriosis, had surgery, and then went on to have three babies. Never mind that every case is different. Never mind that not one of the anecdotes I heard ever involved a woman whose disease was similar to mine. That didn't stop anyone from telling me all the "encouraging" details.

This scenario doesn't play out just among people with endometriosis, of course. It seems as if everyone knows someone who struggled for ten years to conceive and now has a whole houseful of little miracle children. Such stories might be inspiring the first few times you hear one, but after that, they begin to get a little tiresome.

Questions about family status also can be disconcerting. A lady at church once asked me if I had children. When I said no, she replied, "Oh, so you're not married?"

"Do you have a family?" is another common inquiry that can send an infertile person over an emotional cliff. So are "When are you going to start a family?" and "Why don't you have any kids?"

Encouragement following a miscarriage can be particularly brutal. I don't know which is worse—"At least you know your baby is in heaven," "At least you know you can get pregnant," or "You can always try again."

Advice and opinions about various infertility treatments and assisted reproductive procedures also flow freely. If your friends and family members aren't cautioning you against "playing God," and exhorting you to "just have faith," they're pestering you about how long it's taking you to start intervention, reminding you that "you're not getting any younger," or (in the case of parents) bemoaning the fact that they don't have any grandchildren yet.

And then there are all those pat one-liners that people are so fond of tossing out in their attempts to help.

"Just relax."

"Stop trying so hard."

"God is in control."

"I just know God is going to give you a baby."

"Maybe it's not God's will for you to have a baby."

"If it's meant to be, it will happen."

"You can always adopt."

We could probably go on all day and still not plumb the depths of the dumb things people say when they think they're being encouraging. The primary issue isn't whether or not you'll ever be on the receiving end of such remarks and questions—you will. The most significant matter—the factor that can have a huge impact on your emotional and spiritual health—is how you choose to respond to what friends, family members, and strangers say to you about your infertility. I'm not just talking about your verbal responses, although those are very important. I'm also referring to your internal responses—your attitudes, thoughts, and feelings about the words that are said *and* about the people who say them.

Whenever I talk to other women who have experienced infertility at some point in their lives, we nearly always end up comparing notes about this subject at some point in the conversation. It seems to be a fact of life for people who are having trouble getting pregnant, a cross we have to bear as long as we interact with other human beings. But somehow, there's comfort in knowing that other people also have to put up with all those same insensitive comments and silly questions. I hope you have at least one friend with whom you can commiserate about such things. That goes a long way toward relieving the irritation these comments can bring out in even the most patient, tenderhearted person.

Commiseration is not the principal purpose of this chapter, however. Rather, I want to offer some reality-based guidance about how to handle other people and the things that they say. We usually can't control what people say to us. The only thing we can control is how we respond. This is true in every area of life, but it is especially relevant when it comes to infertility. We can take each and every bit of off-the-cuff advice or pat answer personally—which usually leads to anger, bitterness, resentment, and other unhealthy emotions. Or we can take a different approach. It's one that doesn't always ease the pain these statements cause, but one that definitely helps keep our blood pressure down and our peace level up.

By coming at the subject from this angle, you might think that I'm letting the people who make stupid or insensitive comments off the hook. Not so. Appendix A in this book is a guide for friends, family members, and pastors about how to encourage and comfort people who are struggling with infertility. In it, I give straightforward advice about what works and what doesn't work. My goal is to help your loved ones realize how the things they say and do can affect you as you cope with your infertility. At the same time, however, I realize that they may not be open to such instruction. This makes what I'm about to say in this chapter even more important. I repeat: You can't control what other people say, but you can control how you respond. And the first step is trying to understand *why* people say what they say.

The Story Behind the Words

I don't make a habit of analyzing every nuance of every word spoken to me. Through the years, however, I have learned to observe people's behavior and recognize that their words don't always tell the whole story about what's going on with them. For example, when someone appears to be unusually angry with me, it could be because I've done something to upset him or her. But it could also mean that the person is really bothered about something else and is simply taking out that hurt or frustration on me, an innocent bystander.

Stated another way, there is nearly always more to someone's words or actions than meets the eye. There's usually an explanation, a missing piece of the puzzle, or a hidden set of circumstances that triggers the negative response. This doesn't excuse angry outbursts, obnoxious behavior, or hurtful comments. But knowing the rest of the story can sometimes make such encounters easier to stomach.

I have also found this type of reasoning to be very helpful in dealing with the comments other people make about infertility, childbearing, families, and so on. Understanding *why* someone might have said something doesn't always remove the sting of the remark (or make me any less inclined to wring his or her neck at the time), but it does make it much easier to let the comment go and not take it personally.

Before I go on, I should point out that, if you tend to hold grudges or if you're readily inclined to take offense at things and then stew over them for weeks, you might want to skip to the next chapter. What I'm about to say doesn't allow for any of that. Sure, the offense may seem to justify a grudge. But it's simply not worth the emotional and mental strain. You only hurt yourself when you allow things to fester, and the last thing you need when you're struggling with infertility is another source of pain.

Plain Old Insensitivity

That said, let's come up with some reasons to explain why the people around us seem to say the darnedest things about our infertility. First, we have to realize that some people are just insensitive clods. That's all there is to it. They like to spout off all their wisdom, and they don't give a hoot about how their words will make anyone feel. From these people, advice like "You can always adopt" is a stinging slap in the face because you know they're just saying it to hear themselves talk.

It's not always the case, but these people also tend to be extremely self-absorbed—their world is all about them and their problems and stories. They simply don't have the time or the inclination to give you and your life more than a passing glance. If you do happen to make the mistake of telling them something personal, they either ignore it or barely acknowledge it in their haste to turn the focus back on themselves.

It seems as if everyone knows someone who struggled for ten years to conceive and now has a whole houseful of little miracle children.

It's bad enough when such a person has no experience with infertility. But when the offender happens to be half of a barren couple, it's ten times worse. I will never forget what one such person said upon learning the cause of our infertility: "Endometriosis? Yeah, yeah…been there, done that."

If Randy and I hadn't heard this remark with our own ears, we would have never believed that this person had actually said it. We were speechless, to put it mildly. Even now, it makes me cringe to think that someone in his shoes could be so completely lacking in empathy. Of all people, he should have known better than to say something like that. The fact that he did say it was a strong indication to us that he wasn't the most sensitive person in the world.

Self-appointed prophets who are convinced they have all the spiritual answers to your situation also fall into the "insensitive clod" category. In their self-righteous opinion, you're having trouble getting pregnant because you have some kind of sin in your life. If you confess and repent from your sin, perhaps God will have mercy on you and allow you to conceive. They may not tell you all this in so many words, of course. But their attitude around you gives away their true feelings on the subject.

Ignorance is NOT Bliss

We all have friends, relatives, and co-workers who fit the "insensitive clod" description. But I think that most people truly do mean well when they try to comfort and encourage us. They really do think they're being helpful. Unfortunately, many times they are totally ignorant about infertility and the impact it can have on a person mentally, emotionally, physically, and spiritually. They think that because they know someone who had a hard time getting pregnant or they read a newspaper article about infertility, they are equipped to discuss the topic intelligently. In reality, however, they don't have a clue what they're talking about.

Advice such as "just relax," for example, reveals a complete lack of understanding of the physical causes of infertility. As I noted before, in my case, no amount of relaxing could have eliminated the adhesions, scar tissue, and endometriosis that prevented my reproductive organs from working correctly. On a deeper level, pat answers such as "you can always adopt" fail to address all the painful questions and issues that not being able to conceive brings up in a person's life. People who make statements like that don't realize that adoption—as wonderful as it is—will not automatically erase all the physical pain, the theological confusion, and the emotional distress that infertility causes. In their ignorance, they think that the lack of a baby is your most serious problem—one that can easily be fixed through adoption or some high-tech procedure. They don't realize that in addition to an empty nursery, you're also dealing with unmet expectations, the loss of dreams, varying degrees of physical suffering, questions about God's will, doubts about your faith, and so on.

"Helpfulness"

Insensitivity and ignorance aren't the only culprits, of course. Many people make comments that might hurt or annoy us because they just don't know what to say and they haven't learned that it's okay not to say anything at all. Think about this for a minute: How would you react if a friend told you that she had just been diagnosed with breast cancer, or that her father had just been killed in a car accident, or that her husband was having an affair with his secretary? Chances are, you wouldn't know what to say. And rather than deal with an uneasy silence, you just might end up blurting out something you immediately wish you could take back.

This hypothetical situation might give you some idea of what runs through people's minds when they learn you're having trouble getting pregnant. Let's face it—infertility is not the most comfortable subject to discuss, especially if the person you're talking to is noticeably distraught about her circumstances. There are a few wonderful souls in this world who do know how to respond in such situations. Some are just naturally compassionate, while others have allowed the suffering in their own lives to teach them how to empathize. More often than not, however, people just don't know what to say. And so they often end up saying the wrong thing.

Friends and loved ones also say dumb things about conception and infertility because it makes *them* feel better about your condition. It's much easier to tell you "I just know you're going to get pregnant soon" than it is to deal with the possibility that you might not ever conceive. Rattling off Romans 8:28 or repeating some famous quote about God's timing helps them avoid the more troubling questions that infertility often triggers.

Along the same lines, people desperately want everything to be okay for you. So they sometimes make comments that are meant to encourage but fail to take into account the reality of the situation. This hit home with me when my older sister was pregnant with her third baby. Because her first two pregnancies had ended in miscarriages, she was trying very hard to not get her hopes up with the third one, even though everything seemed to be going well. When I found out she was pregnant, I really wanted to reassure her by saying, "I'm sure the baby will be okay," but somehow, those words seemed empty and hollow. I had no idea if the baby was going to be okay or not. I could hope that the child would be fine. I could pray that things would turn out differently this time. But I simply could not tell her "I'm sure everything will be okay" when her past experience suggested the opposite might happen. Such an attempt at comfort would have fallen on deaf ears, and rightly so.

In this case, I knew what my sister had been through and I understood that her fears about losing another baby were not unfounded. I'm sure I didn't always say the right thing, but I was at least aware of what I was saying when I tried to encourage her. Unfortunately, most people either don't know the whole situation or they don't think through all the ramifications of their words before they speak them, which is why comments that are intended to ease your pain often have the reverse effect.

Other times, friends and loved ones simply don't understand where you are in your infertility journey. Instead of helping, which is what they want to do, their words simply annoy. I remember feeling this way after my third surgery, when my chances of getting pregnant were growing slimmer by the day. I was beginning to adjust to the reality that I might never have a biological child, but the people around me were still telling me stories about people they knew who got pregnant after many years of infertility. "It could still happen," they'd say hopefully, not realizing I was secretly wishing they would can the optimism once and for all. "I know it *can* happen," I wanted to holler at them, "but it's starting to look like it's not going to for me, and I need to learn to accept that and get on with my life!"

An Incomplete View of God

As I moved toward releasing my dream of having a biological child, I noticed that some people I talked to were not quite so willing to embrace what I was learning to accept. As I thought about this, it occurred to me that holding on to the hope that I could still get pregnant just might be helping these people avoid a side of God that they really didn't want to face.

Let me explain what I mean. Remember all those theological misconceptions we covered in chapters two and three? *Children are the ultimate sign of God's approval and blessing. Infertility is some kind of divine punishment. If we can't conceive it's because we don't have enough faith. God doesn't really care about those intricate details of our life.* And so on. I hope you now understand what the Bible really says about all that. But unless the people in your life have gone through similar considerations, they may be operating under the same false assumptions that might have troubled you before you found out the truth.

For example, they might believe that it's God's will for all Christians to have biological children. Or if we pray and trust hard enough, God will always give us what we want. When your continued prayers for a child are not answered with a pregnancy, it upsets their preconceived notion of who God is and how He works. They might see you doing all the "right" things—the things that they think would make you an ideal candidate for parenthood in God's eyes—and they can't figure out why God's not responding like they think He should. They certainly don't want to entertain the idea that His plan for your life might not include biological children. When you start talking about that possibility, it makes them extremely uncomfortable. It's much easier for them to keep on wishing than it is to confront the notion that a loving God might have some other plan for you.

There are probably other reasons why people feel compelled to give advice, ask nosy questions, and offer "comforting" words of encouragement. The main thing to keep in mind, though, is that most people really do mean well, even if their efforts fall far short in our eyes. Of course, that can be tough to remember when you're smarting from the sting of a prying inquiry or trying to reorganize your face after you receive a particularly jaw-dropping bit of wisdom. So it helps to formulate a game plan for how you're going to respond to such comments and questions—*before* they come up in a conversation.

A Gracious Response Strategy

Let's start with how to handle the insensitive clods in your life...those wonderful people who always seem to say the wrong thing without regard for how it makes you feel. Chances are, you'll know who fits into this group even before they find out you're having trouble conceiving. Thus the best plan of action is to stay away from them. That's right—don't allow yourself to be put into a situation where you might have to have a lengthy conversation with them.

Of course, that's not always possible or advisable. Such a person may happen to be your mother, your brother, your Sunday school teacher, or your best friend's spouse. In that case, the only appropriate response is to understand that that's just how they are, and that they're not likely going to change. If you *expect* them to make ignorant, insensitive comments about your infertility, at least you'll be somewhat prepared when the inevitable happens. Thinking of some kind of standard, gracious, nonemotional response—such as a simple smile and nod—ahead of time can also help.

What about the rest of the people who cross your path? The key to a healthy response lies in figuring out when you should use such comments as an opportunity to educate someone about infertility versus when you just need to bite your tongue or quickly change the subject. In other words, you need to learn how to pick your battles.

Thinking of some kind of standard, gracious, nonemotional response ahead of time can also help.

For example, I was once part of a Bible study that involved several women I didn't know. During one of our breaks, I was visiting with a few new friends when the subject of children came up (as it often does in such situations). I told them Randy and I were in the process of adopting our first child. They expressed their congratulations, and then one of them then proceeded to tell me about a woman she knew who had adopted a child and then gotten pregnant. The other chimed in with a similar story, and the two of them sat there and carried on a conversation about how wonderful that was, and how adopting a child makes people relax more, which helps them get pregnant, and on and on.

I just sat there between them, not saying a word. I suppose I could have interrupted and informed them that pregnancy after adoption occurs in only 5 percent of such cases,[1] that Randy and I were neither hoping nor expecting it to happen in our family, and that by even bringing it up, they were making it seem as if my beautiful little girl from China was some kind of consolation prize. But I chose to remain silent because they were happy with their conversation. And I could tell that being adamant about the facts wouldn't accomplish anything.

On the other hand, if a close friend or relative had been the one to tell me a story about someone getting pregnant after infertility treatment or adoption, I would have been much more inclined to present the other side of the story. In fact, I took this approach with my mother. After listening to her relay several stories about people who had gotten pregnant after being treated for endometriosis, I finally asked her to stop sharing such reports with me. I wasn't rude or disrespectful. I simply told her that such anecdotes were not helpful and that I didn't want to hear them anymore. My mom, who had had no idea that these stories bothered me, was very understanding when I told her how I felt. To this day, she has been very good about keeping such success tales to herself, and I am very grateful for that.

You might not have the kind of relationship with your mother, mother-in-law, or sister that easily facilitates that kind of discussion. But you may have to spend a lot of time with people who tend to make insensitive remarks about your infertility. In such cases, you owe it to yourself and to your sanity to tell them how you feel about their comments. Speaking up isn't easy, especially for people who aren't used to making waves. But when your emotional well-being—and maybe even a treasured relationship—is at stake, you might need to just bite the bullet and learn to be assertive.

Let's say you have a couple of pregnant friends who like to complain about how sick and tired they are and how fat they're getting. Perhaps they just like to moan and groan. Or maybe they think that by pointing out all the negative aspects of pregnancy, they will make you feel better about not being able to conceive. What they fail to realize is that you would gladly throw up every morning and be exhausted by three o'clock every afternoon if it meant that, in seven or eight months, you would be able to give birth to a biological child. In this situation, you have three options. You could keep your mouth shut, become bitter, and eventually stop hanging around your friends. You could say nothing and make up your mind that your friends' comments are not going to upset you. Or you could figure out some way to gently let your friends know how much their remarks hurt you. The choice is yours.

Obviously, you should avoid the first option. Beyond that, you have to decide which alternative works best for your situation and personality. The only thing you need to remember is, if you choose not to talk to your friends about this problem, you relinquish your right to complain about it. We're dealing with reality here, remember? I know you weren't given a choice about your infertility—none of us were. But you can either turn yourself into a victim who takes offense at every wrong word, or you can allow your circumstances to make you more assertive, more gracious, or more patient with others.

Setting Boundaries

Now that I've established my case for speaking up, I should add that, if you do choose to address the issue, you need to be aware that it might not do any good. Your friends or relatives might not be able to understand where you're coming from. Or they may be so sure their words of wisdom are correct that they keep bringing them up, time and time again. You can't do much about these people once they know you are having trouble getting pregnant. You might, however, be able to avoid some uncomfortable conversations by setting boundaries early on about what you're going to say about your infertility—and to whom you're going to say it.

Some people who are having trouble getting pregnant want to keep their problem a secret from everyone. Some want to tell everyone they know. Others fall somewhere in the middle. Personally, I think it's wise to limit the number of people who know.

When you are having difficulty conceiving, it's tempting to share your pain with others, or to explain the whole sad story when someone asks you if you have any children. But as I pointed out earlier, the more people you confide in and the more information you provide, the more questions you have to deal with during times when you may not feel like answering any questions.

A friend of mine found this out the hard way. She was scheduled to have a blood test done during a month when her husband was out of the country. She had told some friends about the test, and she knew they would be waiting to hear the results. But the further she got into her cycle, the more she began to feel as if her system was somehow out of kilter that month, perhaps due to her husband's absence. She began debating whether she should put the test off until the following month when her husband was home and her schedule had returned to normal. Her health insurance doesn't cover infertility expenses, and she didn't want to spend the money to have the test done only to have the results skewed due to a one-time disruption in her system. At the same time, she felt she owed her friends an explanation. But she didn't want to have to tell them she had put off the test another month.

This experience taught my friend that it's often best to keep such tests and procedures private—or share them only with a few close friends who also are dealing with fertility problems. There is such a thing as too much information, especially when it comes to infertility. You're not obligated to keep anyone up-to-date about your progress (or lack thereof). If friends or relatives ask, you have every right to limit what you tell them, if you tell them anything.

That said, I also would caution against going to the other extreme of keeping your infertility a secret from everyone. In the first place, it's far too difficult of a trial to handle alone. You really need the support and prayers of a few trusted friends to help you endure it. Secondly, keeping it to yourself can lead you down a path of deception that might help you retain your privacy but will do absolutely nothing to enhance your peace level. If you choose not to tell your parents that you're seeing a specialist, for example, you might be setting yourself up for a situation in which you have to lie about everything from doctor appointments to why you can't go out to dinner on a night when you need to be at home trying to conceive.

Lying is a sin, no matter what the reason. Don't put yourself in a position where you are constantly worrying about how you are going to explain why you don't feel well or why you've been to the doctor. Rather, come up with a plan for telling your closest loved ones at least a few sketchy details. I realize that informing your parents or other relatives that you're having trouble getting pregnant might open the door to all kinds of conversations you'd rather avoid. One solution to this tricky scenario might be to sit down with your parents and say something like, "We wanted you to know that we're trying to get pregnant, but we're having some trouble. We're seeing an infertility specialist, and he's doing everything he can to find out what's wrong. We just want you to know so we don't have to lie about what we're doing. This is very difficult, and we don't really want to talk about it a whole lot right now, so we'd appreciate it if you would just keep us in your prayers and not ask us about it. We'll keep you posted if there's something you need to know."

If the very thought of having a conversation like this with your mother makes you break out in hives, you might want to consider writing a letter. Whatever route you take, the key is to be honest about what you're going through, without feeling the need to explain it all or discuss things you'd prefer to keep to yourself. This might require you to be far more assertive than you've ever been before. In the long run, though, it will be worth it because it will give you a bit of control over discussions about your infertility.

Like Water off a Duck's Back

In a perfect world, there would be no need for a chapter like this. None of your friends, relatives, neighbors, or co-workers would ever utter an insensitive word, and they'd always be completely understanding of how your infertility affects you. Of course, in a perfect world, this whole book would be unnecessary, because there would be no such thing as infertility. Such a place doesn't exist this side of heaven, however. So if you want to retain your sanity as you try to get pregnant, you basically have to develop a very thick skin.

I know it's not fair. I don't like putting up with nosy and insensitive people any more than you do. But no matter where you are in your infertility journey, and regardless of how that journey eventually ends, you simply must learn to let things go. It's very tempting to hold a perpetual pity party for yourself. But you simply can't take all those ignorant, thoughtless, or unkind comments to heart—because they *will* plant seeds of bitterness and anger deep within your soul that will be difficult to dig out later.

I'm not saying you shouldn't express distress or even anger at the stupid things people say to you. As I mentioned before, sharing them with your spouse or with other infertile friends is a good way to get them off your chest so you don't internalize them. Randy and I often swap such stories, and we nearly always end up having a good laugh at the absurdity of the whole situation, whatever it is.

Telling God how you feel about such conversations also helps. If you're fed up with everyone else's opinions and feel like clubbing the next person who offers you some useless bit of advice, ask God to give you the grace, wisdom, and kindness you need to respond. Ask Him to help you love the people around you even when they're not even trying to understand what you're going through. Most importantly, ask Him to show you ways that you can minister to the very people whose words are causing you so much grief. By doing so, you will "heap burning coals" on their heads, as Proverbs 25:22 so eloquently puts it. The insensitive words may not stop, but God will reward you for your efforts and attitude.

Once you've got your thick skin in place, you can start evaluating your own empathy levels when it comes to the suffering of other people. When someone says something insensitive to you—tuck it away in a mental file labeled "things I should never say to someone who is hurting." Instead of letting ignorant comments and pat answers harden your heart, allow them to make your heart softer and more in tune with the feelings of others.

This is what my friend who was feeling obligated to keep everyone updated about her fertility progress has done. She was tremendously kindhearted to begin with, but being forced to deal with difficult comments about her fertility problems has made her much more aware of what she says when she's trying to encourage others, no matter what their suffering involves. This heightened awareness has been a valuable tool for my friend, because she is a pastor's wife and often has the opportunity to interact with hurting people. But it's not just beneficial for people in ministry—it's a positive lesson we all can learn from our infertility experience, no matter what our profession or calling in life.

As far as I'm concerned, few things are sadder than a person who goes through infertility and fails to use the journey as a tool to sharpen his or her own sensitivity skills. It just seems like such a waste of a good trial. I don't know about you, but if I have to go through something painful, I prefer to make the experience as productive as possible. If there are lessons to be learned from it, I like to learn them the first time so I don't have to repeat the course later. I don't know if I've completed my sensitivity training yet, but I am much more conscious of what I say to people who are coping with divorce, serious illnesses, family difficulties, and other problems than I used to be. And I try not to say anything to someone else that I would not want to hear myself.

I slip up every now and then, but that's all part of the growth process. A thick skin doesn't develop without some degree of battering, and a soft heart isn't created without any tears. But when both exist in the same person, they allow for a degree of strength and compassion that is hard to find in someone who has never experienced any kind of suffering.

Remember that the next time someone encourages you to "just relax."

EIGHT

A Slightly Different Approach to Infertility Treatment

In my life, September has never stood out as a particularly eventful month. It's usually unbearably hot and humid where I live, my flowerbeds look pathetic, and I'm still weeks away from celebrating my birthday or any other favorite holidays. If you factor out the horrible events of September 11, 2001 (which I admit is difficult to do), the ninth month of our family's calendar year simply isn't very interesting or memorable.

And yet, when it comes to my infertility journey, I'll not soon forget what happened in late September 2000. A few weeks earlier, Randy and I had gone to the doctor for what we had decided would be our third and final attempt at intrauterine insemination (IUI). As usual, the wait for results had been somewhat nerve-racking. (Though this time, a short business trip to Los Angeles had kept my mind occupied for a few of those days.)

As the date when I normally would start my period approached, I began to wonder if this might be *the* month. In three years of trying to conceive, I remember missing only one period, and that was due to surgery, not to cyclical irregularities or possible pregnancy. I had never even been late—not one single time. So when the twenty-seventh day of my cycle came and went without any of the usual telltale signs, I began to get my hopes up. I even did something I had never done before. I went to the store and bought a pregnancy test.

I took the test on the evening of the twenty-eighth day. The box said to wait longer, but I wasn't about to let what could be my last chance to take a pregnancy test slip by without capitalizing on it. Anxious excitement gripped Randy and me as we set the timer for the required wait. When the bell went off, we entered the bathroom and nervously peeked at the results.

The test was negative.

Not ready to give up just yet, I decided to call the doctor's office in the morning and see if the nurse had any words of wisdom for me. She did. Home pregnancy tests aren't reliable, she told me. If I hadn't started in a week, I was to come in for a blood test, which would accurately indicate whether or not I was pregnant.

I'd never gone 29 days without a period, and I took this as a very positive sign. I shared my hopes with a friend over lunch—but even then, my body was starting to send out the familiar signals that my period was on its way.

A few hours later, we had our answer. The IUI had failed. I wasn't pregnant.

Even more significant was the fact that our intentional efforts to conceive were officially over. We hadn't done all we could have done, but we had done all we wanted to do. It was time to stop.

I don't recollect much of what happened next. I know we were extremely disappointed and incredibly sad, and I'm sure there were some tears involved. But we really weren't devastated, even though such a reaction would have been totally understandable. If anything, one of the feelings I most remember was that of relief...that these agonizing waits were over, that I wouldn't have to go back to the doctor for any more uncomfortable procedures or tests, that I could stop being an infertility patient and get on with my life.

About six months earlier, I had been recovering from my third major surgery for severe endometriosis. As I explained earlier, the aggressive nature of my disease had prompted the doctor who performed the surgery to strongly urge us to consider in vitro fertilization, either immediately (his recommendation) or after no more than three or four IUI attempts that had little chance of succeeding. So how did Randy and I go from hearing that IVF was our only real hope to closing the door to any further treatment, all in six months' time? What made us decide not to move on to in vitro fertilization after three IUI attempts? And if we really wanted a biological baby, why did we decide to stop trying to get pregnant after only three years?

Overwhelmed by the Options

The answers to those questions aren't simple. Neither are the issues that Christian couples who are struggling with infertility need to work through as they make decisions about how far they're willing to go in their own efforts to conceive. Reproductive science has advanced a great deal in recent years, and infertile couples have many more medical options than they had in previous generations. These include sophisticated diagnostic testing, potent fertility drugs, and an array of procedures that fall under the heading of *assisted reproductive technology* (ART). This basically means that those procedures involve the "manipulation of human eggs and/or sperm for the purpose of establishing a pregnancy."[1]

These options have enabled many people to have children. But in some ways, because of all the difficult choices involved, they also have increased the anguish of infertility. Not only do people have to think about which treatment alternatives are ethically acceptable, they also have to decide which ones they actually want to pursue, how many cycles to attempt, and how much money they're willing to invest in ventures with unsure out-comes. Committed Christian couples have the added pressure of trying to discern how all these high-tech medical solutions fit into God's specific plan for them.

Your chief aim right now might be to get pregnant. There's nothing wrong with that. But the choices you make to achieve that outcome could have ramifications—and perhaps consequences—that will affect you long after the baby (or babies, as the case may be) arrives. You owe it to yourself, your spouse, *and* your future children to equip yourself to make choices you won't regret later.

We hadn't done all we could have done, but we had done all we wanted to do. It was time to stop.

Nearly every infertility book and article I've read contains numerous testimonies from people—conscientious, committed Christian people—who, in their desperate attempts to get preg-nant, tried one costly procedure after another until they had frit-tered away their entire savings and several years of their lives. Often they had nothing to show for it. I really don't think most of these people planned to do this when they first realized they had a fertility problem—it just kind of happened.

In our society, when you realize you are having trouble getting pregnant, you might deny it at first. Then you might fret about it for a few months (maybe longer) and after that go to your gynecologist to find out what's wrong. Unless you have a history of medical problems, "finding out what's wrong" usually begins with a physical exam. This is generally followed by instructions to take your basal body temperature every morning or monitor ovulation with a store-bought predictor kit for several months. Next come blood work, postcoital tests, semen analyses, ultrasounds, cervical-mucus evaluations, and, if nothing turns up, perhaps an endometrial biopsy, hysterosalpingogram (an X ray of the uterus and fallopian tubes, also known as an HSG), or diagnostic laparoscopy.

If a problem is detected, the first step of treatment might involve fertility drugs, which are often prescribed to correct hormonal imbalances. If the medication doesn't achieve the desired result, at some point, either you or your gynecologist may decide it's time for you to see an infertility specialist. One thing leads to another, and—if everything else fails—before you know it, you and your spouse are sitting in the specialist's office, listening to him explain your chances with IUI, IVF, or any number of other mysterious-sounding abbreviations.

Responsible Decisions

By the point you're talking with the specialist, you might feel as if you're backed into a corner with no choice but to follow his recommendations. He's the expert, after all. When he utters those famous words "Our goal is to get you pregnant," followed by a plan of action, who are you to argue? Truth be told, you almost feel obligated to try every available medical recourse—for as long as it takes to "get you pregnant." God gave doctors the wisdom and ability to come up with all these procedures, didn't He? So doesn't that mean you should try them all until one works?

Not necessarily.

Just because the technology exists doesn't mean you have to use it. That's the simple truth. I'm not saying that Christians should never pursue aggressive medical treatment for infertility. I am saying, however, that you are not required to do so. You might be feeling pressure from yourself, your extended family, your doctors, your friends, and even society at large to hurry up and do everything you can to conceive a child. But you cannot base your decisions on what other people think, because ultimately, you are not responsible to them for your actions. You are responsible to God. And someday you will stand before Him and give an account for your life—including what you did with your time and how you used the resources with which you were entrusted. This account will certainly cover the years that you devoted to trying to get pregnant. They won't be exempted because you were going through such a difficult trial. As a result, the choices you make regarding your infertility treatment are extremely important, not just because they may affect whether or not you are able to conceive, but also because they are a direct reflection of your priorities and motives.

This is not an easy topic to discuss. It's very difficult to write about because I know what a sensitive issue it is. After all, those who elect not to pursue medical treatment feel strongly about their decision. So do those who choose to try ARTs such as in vitro fertilization (which involves "removing eggs from a woman, fertilizing them in a culture dish...and later transferring the embryo[s] into the uterus"[2]), gamete intrafallopian transfer (GIFT, where egg and sperm are retrieved, then mixed in the fallopian tubes), zygote intrafallopian transfer (ZIFT, where a single-cell embryo called a *zygote* is transferred to the fallopian tubes before it divides[3]), intracytoplasmic sperm injection (ISCI, which involves injecting a single sperm into one egg), or various surrogacy arrangements.

This whole subject can make people extremely defensive because it involves very personal decisions that are often criticized by third parties who don't know anything about infertility. The truth of the matter is, however, that godly people have different opinions about what is acceptable and what is not when it comes to helping conception to occur. What you decide to do is between you, your spouse, your doctor, and God. I do want to share with you, though, what I believe God has called me to write about this subject.

Go Ahead, But Set Boundaries

I don't think Christians should take a totally hands-off approach to infertility. I encourage friends who are having difficulty conceiving to do whatever they can to determine the cause of the problem, as long as they realize that even the most sophisticated testing may not result in a clear diagnosis. Some may choose not to do this, and I respect that decision. But for many people, including me, not knowing what's wrong can be excruciatingly difficult. Undergoing diagnostic tests can alleviate some of the stress and worry that accompany the ambiguity. Of course, conclusive test results can trigger a whole new batch of emotions and fears, but at least you have a better idea of what you're up against.

The testing phase can take several months. This gives you a great opportunity to research all the treatment options and come up with a game plan for what you'd be willing to try if your infertility cannot be resolved easily. This might sound like an odd suggestion. After all, each test is accompanied by hope that it might be the one to identify a correctable problem. But this is really the best time to develop your infertility treatment "philosophy" because you are still able to be somewhat objective about the options. It's much easier to set boundaries about what you're willing to do when you're undergoing testing. If you wait until the doctor tells you that artificial insemination by donor (AID) is your only option, then you have to endure the stress of trying to decide whether that procedure is right for you at a time when you are especially vulnerable emotionally.

It's similar to setting boundaries in any other area of life. You don't wait until a stranger is flirting with you at the airport to decide if you're going to remain faithful to your spouse—if you're wise, you made that choice before you got married, and the gold band on your hand is an ever-present reminder of your commitment. Such boundaries, whether they involve fidelity or infertility, are never established in the heat of the moment. If they are, they usually don't hold. They must be established ahead of time, thoughtfully and prayerfully, so they can protect your heart and provide a solid foundation for you to stand on when you are faced with a difficult choice.

You owe it to yourself, your spouse, and your future children to equip yourself to make choices you won't regret later.

As you're doing your research and formulating your strategy, think through all the worst-case scenarios and evaluate all the possible solutions to those situations. What if the problem is an extremely low sperm count? Would you be willing to consider AID? What are the pros and cons of such a choice? What are the moral and relational ramifications of using a third party's sperm to conceive a child? Assume you can't get pregnant because your fallopian tubes are severely damaged. What do you think about IVF? Consider the physical risks, the possibility of multiple births, the cost, and the ethical implications.

Go through this type of exercise with every infertility treatment and ART you read about in magazine articles, books (both Christian and secular), and on reputable Internet sites (see appendix C for some recommended resources). Evaluate all the options through the lens of a biblical worldview, never forgetting that life begins at conception, whether that conception occurs in a petri dish or a woman's uterus. If you need help with any of this, talk to your pastor or a trusted spiritual mentor—someone who is able to think through issues carefully without making snap judgments.

Once you've done all this, compare notes with your spouse and put your thoughts on paper. You obviously can't decide exactly what you're going to do because you lack the medical expertise to make such decisions on your own. Plus, you're still waiting to find out why you can't get pregnant. You can, however, come up with a clearly defined set of boundaries. These boundaries will make clear where you will draw the line when it comes to ARTs. They will specify the maximum length of time or number of cycles you will devote to trying to get pregnant. In other words, you can put down what you *won't* do and set a deadline for how long you're going to try. Such decisions aren't necessarily set in stone, but neither should they be viewed as completely optional. That would defeat the purpose of what you're doing.

Lay the Groundwork for Good Decisions

I realize an exercise like this can be overwhelming, discouraging, and even depressing. When you're trying to figure out why you're having trouble conceiving, the last thing you want to think about is the possibility that you might not be able to produce a child without some high-tech medical procedure—one that seems as if it came straight off the pages of a science-fiction novel. Nor do you want to contemplate the idea that you could be spending the next several years of your life trying to have a baby. But if you don't think through these things on the front end, you could wake up one day and wonder where the last six years went and why you allowed yourself to pursue all those procedures that you really weren't comfortable with. That's what we want to avoid.

You might feel some discouragement while you do your research and wait for test results. To combat this, consistently pray for the grace and strength to accept God's plan for your life, regardless of whether that plan includes a biological child. Use what you learned in chapter four as a guide. Diligently remind God of your desire for a baby. Pour out your heart to Him when you're feeling despondent, impatient, or angry. But always include some variation of Christ's prayer in the garden of Gethsemane—"Not my will, but yours be done" (Luke 22:42).

When you pray this way, you lay the groundwork that will enable you to make the right choices about your infertility treatment. I don't know how or why this happens. I'll leave such explanations to theologians with years of seminary training. All I know is that in some inexplicable way, praying like this opens the door for the peace of God to take control of your heart and serve as the gatekeeper for every decision you make as you travel along the path of infertility.

Without the help of this divine gatekeeper, you might still accidentally choose the right options. But you will constantly second-guess yourself and wonder if you're doing the right thing. On the other hand, when you commit the outcome of your childbearing efforts to God, establish boundaries that are in keeping with your biblical and ethical convictions, and consistently bathe the whole process in prayer, you might not always like or enjoy the choices you are called to make...but you will have peace about them.

NINE

Joining God

$$\sim\!\!\sim\!\!\sim$$

*B*y now you may be thinking, *Okay, all this stuff about boundaries and infertility-treatment strategies sounds nice in theory, but does it actually work? Is it really possible to set limits and stick to them? And does all that stuff about God's peace really make much difference in real life?*

My answer to all of these questions is a resounding *yes*. But I'm not just going to leave it at that. I'd like to give you an up-close-and-personal glimpse of the questions Randy and I asked ourselves and the factors we considered as we decided what our limits were. Up to this point, all you know is that we decided not to do in vitro fertilization (IVF) even though the doctor said it was our only realistic option. Now I'm going to tell you why. And I'll give you more things to think about as you contemplate your infertility treatment strategy.

Money Matters

Let's start off with a relatively straightforward issue: money. Just about the first thing you learn from your doctor, in your research, and from listening to your friends who have sought medical help for infertility, is this: Attempting to get pregnant can be very expensive. It might seem crass to evaluate an intimate issue like conceiving a child from an economic standpoint, but for Randy and me, money was an important consideration.

As I said before, our health insurance doesn't cover infertility expenses. So any money we spent on trying to get pregnant had to come straight out of our own pockets. We don't have access to a large stock portfolio or a hefty bank account, but we both believe in the importance of saving for a rainy day and investing for future expenses such as our own retirement and college for our children. We began putting money away for college expenses before we even started trying to get pregnant. And we weren't opposed to using some, though not all, of those funds in our efforts to expand our family.

Basically, we had to decide whether paying $8000 or $9000 for an IVF attempt was the best use of our financial resources. We had the money, but were we willing to spend it on a procedure that has less than a 40 percent chance of working? What if it didn't work the first time? Would we have the strength to stop? Or would we be tempted to spend another $9000 on a second or third try (maybe even more)?

We're both fairly conservative when it comes to money. So although we really wanted a baby, we simply weren't comfortable putting that much of our hard-earned savings into something when we couldn't be assured of a positive outcome. We believe the Bible calls us to be good stewards of the resources with which we have been entrusted. We felt, therefore, that it would be much better stewardship to put that money toward the cost of an international adoption, which we felt would be much more likely to result in an actual child for our family.

You might be in our situation. Or you might be faced with a different set of financial circumstances. When it comes to finances, every couple has a unique set of issues to consider. Some with large disposable incomes might never miss the $10,000, $20,000, or more (often much, much more) that they might spend on ARTs. That doesn't necessarily mean that's how God would want them to use their money, but it might make the financial aspects of infertility treatment less of a concern for them. Some couples are fortunate enough to have health insurance that covers a wide array of infertility expenses. For these people, the decision whether or not to pursue ARTs may be based on other factors. Many others, however, have few savings and no insurance coverage for infertility. This means that, in order to try a procedure such as IVF (or even to pay for diagnostic testing, fertility drugs, or less aggressive procedures), they might have to take out a second mortgage, get a loan from a bank, borrow from friends or family, use a credit card, or work out some kind of payment plan with their doctor.

What if it didn't work the first time? Would we have the strength to stop?

If you fall into this latter category, I would strongly caution you to think long and hard before you go into debt to finance your infertility treatments. Proverbs 22:7 asserts that "the borrower becomes the lender's slave" (NASB). Is your desire for a child so strong that you would be willing to subject yourself to financial slavery in order to fulfill it?

I once read about a woman who was so desperate to continue treatment (after the money ran out, that is) that she went behind her husband's back to secure a couple of new credit cards so they could finance another procedure. (He thought she had borrowed the money from a relative).[1] You may not think you'd ever resort to such tactics to get pregnant, but desperate people do strange things sometimes. No matter what your financial situation, the wise thing to do is to think about how much you can realistically afford to spend on infertility treatment. Then pray about what you can spend and still remain a good steward of your money. After that, set a limit that is agreeable to both you and your spouse, and stick to that limit.

How Is All This Going to Affect Me?

Although it was an important consideration, money wasn't the only factor that influenced our decision not to pursue IVF or let our attempts to get pregnant drag on for an unspecified amount of time. We also were very concerned about the physical, emotional, and relational ramifications of extended infertility treatment. I could devote an entire chapter to this subject, but here I'll just touch on a few things we thought about in regard to how all this treatment was going to affect us personally.

First of all, we had to decide how long we were willing to stay on the emotional roller-coaster ride that accompanies infertility. You know the drill. Every month we'd get our hopes up, only to have them dashed to the ground once again. This monthly process affected me and Randy differently. He would remain hopeful up until the last minute, while I would usually begin to think the worst when my body started sending out signals that I was about to start my period. When that happened, I tended to put all my energy into preparing myself for the physical pain I knew was coming, rather than grieving about the fact that I wasn't pregnant. Looking back, it was probably some kind of defense mechanism, a way of protecting my emotions. Randy, on the other hand, had no such physical warnings. So he often felt the disappointment of not being pregnant more acutely than I did—at least initially.

Although we handled this process differently, we both knew there was a limit to how much of it we could stand, both as a couple and as individuals. By the time we decided to try some intrauterine inseminations (IUIs), we had already been riding on this roller coaster for several years. We'd been trying to get pregnant for most of that time. A good part of it, though, had also been devoted to dealing with medical issues that were related to infertility but also had more serious health implications. Once those problems were resolved, we had to ask ourselves how much more time and emotional energy we wanted to devote to more extensive infertility treatment. That's when we decided we would do no more than three inseminations. After that, we would stop trying to conceive.

We were fortunate that our infertility did not drive a wedge between us and harm our marriage. If anything, it actually brought us closer. But it did affect certain aspects of our relationship. Month after month of planning intimate moments around an ovulation predictor kit can turn an act that is meant to be special into something mechanical, even dreaded at times. We did what we had to do, of course—but I'd be lying if I said I wasn't relieved when we could finally have sex for the sheer pleasure of it, not because we had to. Had it not been for our predetermined stopping point, we might *still* be forcing ourselves to have intercourse on command and getting our hopes up every month.

Effects of Drugs

Our views about fertility drugs also affected our decisions about the types and number of procedures we were willing to try. Many people accept the side effects of these drugs simply as a means to an end. But I have to think very seriously before I take a medication that has the potential to make me sick or turn me into an emotional basket case, regardless of how many eggs it makes my ovaries produce. I won't let a dentist give me laughing gas because I don't like the out-of-control feeling it gives me. So would I really want to take a drug that causes me to be laughing one minute, crying the next, and experiencing a hot flash the next? Not if I can avoid it.

And what about the long-term physical effects of these drugs? Some researchers say women who take fertility drugs have a higher risk of ovarian cancer than the general population, while others say no such risk exists.[2] I took Clomid for a few cycles to give the IUIs a better chance at succeeding. However, I was unwilling to put my future health at risk by taking the stronger drugs necessary for IVF or other procedures that involve egg retrieval. Some people are willing to accept the unknown risks of these drugs if it means they might be able to fulfill their dream of having a biological child. I understand that, but I wasn't one of them. You shouldn't take fertility drugs just because your gynecologist or reproductive endocrinologist prescribes them for you. Read up on them, find out the potential risks and side effects, and *then* decide whether you want to take them.

Speaking of fertility drugs, the possibility of multiple births also was something that we considered in our decisions. The idea of twins was acceptable—even somewhat exciting—to me, but the notion of having three, four, five, or more children at once was more than I could tolerate. For one thing, I didn't know if my body could handle the stress of carrying that many babies. And what if they were all born prematurely? Did we have the emotional and financial resources to deal with possible special needs and potentially life-threatening situations? On the home front, I certainly didn't relish the notion of having to care for multiple newborns. And what would happen as the children grew older? Would I have the energy to love and care for each one in such a way that would help him or her to grow up to be an emotionally healthy, well-adjusted person? Would we be able to handle, mentally and financially, the cost of having several children in diapers, in braces, or leaving for college at the same time?

Now I know there are plenty of people who would love the opportunity to welcome three or four precious little babies into the world at once. Or at least that's what they think when they are having trouble getting pregnant. Unfortunately, the desire to have a child can cloud a person's judgment and make him or her view things like multiple births through rose-colored glasses. I realize that many people who take fertility drugs and try various ARTs do not conceive more than one child, but multiple births are always a possibility. Don't let the romantic notion of being surrounded by several chubby-cheeked cherubs make you forget the long- and short-term reality of the situation. If you think you're up for the challenge, that's great. But don't forge ahead until you've thought through *all* the ramifications.

I could probably go on all day about the physical, emotional, and relational aspects of extended infertility treatment. The more I think about it, however, the more I realize that my answers to many of my questions boiled down to the fact that I'm just not much of a risk-taker. I know it's sometimes worth it to try something, even if you know it might not work. But when it came to infertility treatment, there were some risks I just wasn't willing to take. What if we had tried IVF and it had failed? I don't know if my heart could have withstood that much disappointment and sorrow. I know people deal with it every day, but I just wasn't willing to put myself through that.

Only you know how much you can take. Just keep a couple of things in mind as you think about all this: If your tolerance for risk is similar to mine, you may occasionally feel selfish or foolish for not doing more. If you're more willing to take informed chances, then you'll probably have to deal with uninformed people who question your choices, admonish you to "leave it up to God," or accuse you of trying to "play God."

Ethical Implications

Sadly, such accusations often fly most freely among people who would view themselves as caring, compassionate Christians. Recently I met someone who told me that, when she and her husband were going through infertility treatments, they didn't tell any of their Christian friends what they were doing. Why? They were afraid of being judged unfairly for their decisions. Her comment made me sad because I believe people who are dealing with infertility have a great need for medically sound *and* theologically solid counsel about all their treatment options. And yet, so often all they get is criticism. Or they get advice from people who don't know anything about infertility. Or they get one-sided recommendations from infertility doctors who specialize in ARTs. This is unfortunate, because decisions about infertility treatment absolutely must be thought through from an ethical standpoint. And it can be difficult to do that without input from an objective third party.

In our case, ethical uncertainties played a major role in our decision not to pursue IVF. From the very beginning, Randy had reservations about the procedure. The idea of growing babies in petri dishes seemed a bit too much like science fiction to him. When he mentioned this during one of our initial visits to the infertility clinic, the doctor basically ignored him. That wasn't a big surprise, of course. The doctor makes his living doing IVF, and I'm sure he didn't want to acknowledge that a procedure he does regularly might fall into an ethical gray area, at least in the minds of some people.

Fortunately, we weren't counting on the doctor's guidance to help us decide whether or not we wanted to do in vitro. We had already researched the procedure. And although we knew other godly people who had done it successfully, we had come to the conclusion that it wasn't right for us—long before we met with the doctor.

Some Christians who approve of procedures such as IVF assert that, since God gave the scientists the wisdom to develop ARTs, we are welcome to use them. However, we need to be careful when we use this argument to determine whether some of the procedures are morally justified. I certainly believe that God uses doctors to help sick people get well and infertile women get pregnant. But while man has used his God-given wisdom to develop some very good things, he's also used it to come up with some horribly destructive things. On top of that, technology that is intended to be productive and helpful often leads to other things with not-so-pleasant implications.

Concerns About Certain Procedures

Assisted reproductive technology is a case in point. When scientists developed methods of joining a human egg and sperm outside the womb, they most probably had the honorable intention of wanting to help infertile people have biological children. They have achieved that goal: Since the birth of the world's first test-tube baby in 1978, IVF has allowed thousands of couples to realize their dream of becoming parents.

If the scientists who developed IVF had been content to stop there, we might not be having this discussion—but as is often the case, many were not. As a result, today we're being forced to deal with issues such as embryonic stem-cell research and human cloning—topics that were confined to the pages of futuristic novels only a few decades ago.

I'm not suggesting that a procedure is unethical simply because it might eventually lead to something as horrifying as using helpless and defenseless embryos for medical research. But once I learned how IVF was developed (see Debra Evans' book *Without Moral Limits* for more information on this) and I started reading about what it has led to, my personal reservations about the procedure increased.

This wasn't the only thing relating to IVF that bothered Randy and me. We also were opposed to what is blandly called "selective reduction." This is a procedure sometimes done in the first trimester of a multiple pregnancy in which some of the fertilized embryos are aborted—or "reduced"—to "increase the chances that the remaining babies will be carried to term."[3] And we had significant qualms about cyropreservation, a process in which unused embryos are frozen and stored for possible implantation during another IVF cycle. The thought of freezing a tiny human being for later use made me sick to my stomach. So did the notion of destroying a few lives to give a few more a supposedly better shot at life. In my opinion, both of these practices devalue life and show a tremendous lack of respect for the inherent, God-given worth of every individual, no matter how small.

Only you know how much you can take.

Fortunately, neither selective reduction nor cyropreservation is required for IVF to be successful. Infertility patients can avoid both issues by limiting the number of embryos they allow to be fertilized to the number of babies that they are willing to carry to term. I believe this is an ethically acceptable option, although limiting the number of embryos that are fertilized and then transferred to the uterus also limits the chances that a pregnancy will occur.

As Randy and I thought about all these concerns, we came to the conclusion that we would rather avoid IVF entirely than be forced to make decisions about how many eggs to fertilize, whether or not freezing the extra embryos would be okay, or anything else related to starting life outside the womb. As much as we wanted a baby, we simply didn't want to have to deal with all these issues. To this day, we have peace about saying no to IVF. That is all the proof we need that we made the decision that was right for us.

Others have chosen differently, also without regrets. Take my friends Carey and Scott McNair, for example. After trying to get pregnant for six years, they signed up for an in vitro program in St. Louis. At the time, the IVF waiting list at their infertility clinic was quite long. Since they didn't want to put off expanding their family any longer, they decided to adopt a baby from China.

Shortly after they came home with their daughter, Nikki, the clinic called to say they were next in line for IVF. Carey still wanted the opportunity to experience pregnancy, but she and Scott were enjoying their time with their 6-month-old daughter, so they decided to put off the procedure until the next year. Their plans changed, however, when Scott learned that their health insurance, which was covering 90 percent of infertility-related expenses at the time, was going to reduce that coverage significantly come January. Presented with this new set of circumstances, they decided to go ahead and do IVF. But they proceeded within specific boundaries that they had established after seeking biblical counsel and devoting considerable thought and prayer to the whole situation. Despite their doctor's objections, they chose to have only seven eggs fertilized, three of which became embryos.

Happily, Carey became pregnant with twins, who were born when Nikki was 15 months old. Because of the thought they put into their infertility treatment at the front end, the McNairs can look back at what they did without regrets. They don't have any frozen embryos in a lab somewhere. They didn't put themselves in a position where they would have been forced to choose between carrying quintuplets to term or aborting some of the babies in hopes of helping a few others survive. As a result, they have as much peace about what they chose to do as Randy and I have about what we did.

The Ever-Present Danger of Idolatry

The McNairs' story is encouraging, not only because it had a happy ending, but because it shows what can happen when decisions about infertility treatment are made ahead of time in a thoughtful, rational manner. Unfortunately, many people are unwilling to consider this approach for one simple reason—it would require them to set limits on what they will do to become pregnant. They're so desperate to produce a biological child that they will stop at nothing to achieve that goal.

This attitude is what leads people to apply for credit cards without their spouses' knowledge, spend their entire life's savings on one costly ART after another, set themselves up for multiple pregnancies that could hurt their health and their ability to be good parents, and compromise their previously held convictions about the inherent dignity of human life.

Such actions suggest that the quest to conceive a child has turned into an obsession—or, to put it a little more bluntly, an idol. It might sound a little extreme to suggest that something as honorable as the desire to become a parent could ever turn into something as ugly as an idol. But the danger is very real. And it doesn't even have to involve draining your savings account or deceiving your spouse.

I know this because I experienced it myself. There were times in my infertility journey, primarily in the first year or so, when practically every aspect of my life revolved around getting pregnant. The desire consumed me—to the point where nearly every conversation I had, everything I read, and every church or work activity I participated in left me thinking about having a baby, wondering why it was taking so long, or worrying about what was wrong.

A certain amount of this is normal for someone who is trying to get pregnant. Often there comes a point, though, when getting pregnant becomes the sole focus, and nothing else matters. This type of obsession doesn't happen at once—it grows slowly, never revealing its ultimate intent to displace God at the center of your life. If you're not careful, however, that's exactly what will happen.

You won't wake up one morning and find a little wooden fertility god in the corner of your bedroom. But if you're obsessed with getting pregnant to the point where you have placed your relationship with Christ on the back burner, or if you're single-mindedly pursuing a medical solution to your infertility problem without trusting God to direct your steps, there's a very real chance that you've allowed a graven image to be erected in your heart.

Idolatry is a dangerous business. For one thing, God expressly forbids it (see Exodus 20:3-4), and anytime you willfully violate one of His direct commands, you're asking for trouble. In many situations, desiring something else more than God also leads people to force open doors that should have remained closed. And that inevitably leads to heartache and disappointment.

God's Timetable

The best way to avoid this kind of pain is to wait for God's timing rather than trying to force the issue yourself. But when you're having trouble getting pregnant, that can be a difficult—and very confusing—assignment. For some reason, infertility can make even the most patient believers start trying to make things happen on their own. And even more baffling is the fact that this seems to be expected—even encouraged—by some Christians.

A friend of mine who would like to become a mother was recently asked how long she and her husband had been trying to get pregnant. Upon hearing that they had been trying for about 11 months, the Christian co-workers she was talking to immediately began asking if she had been to the doctor yet and what she and her husband were doing to improve their chances of conceiving. This made my friend very uncomfortable. For one, she is not particularly worried about the fact that she's not pregnant. Neither is she ready to start seeking medical help for what may or may not prove to be an infertility problem.

The way my friend's co-workers reacted to her situation suggests that they don't quite understand that foundational biblical principles—such as trusting God and waiting for His timing—apply to the quest for a child as much as they relate to other life-changing decisions, such as choosing a mate.

Why is it that we encourage single people who long to be married to be patient and wait for God to bring along the right spouse? Yet when someone hasn't gotten pregnant after 11 months, we can't send them to the doctor fast enough! Is human reproduction somehow exempt from biblical teachings on patience, submission, and trust? If not, why are we so eager to take matters into our own hands and put our faith in doctors and technology, instead of in God?

As I stressed in the last chapter, I'm not advocating a hands-off approach to infertility treatment. But I do think that many people who are having trouble conceiving would be much better off in the long run if they waited for God to move—instead of rushing out to seek a medical solution to their problem.

The Old Testament contains some striking case studies of what can happen when someone chooses to wait for God's timing. David, for example, refused to force his career, even when that seemed like the most logical course of action. After all, God, through the prophet Samuel, had told David that he was going to be the next king of Israel. If I had been in David's sandals, I might have spent the next several years strategizing about how I was going to peacefully take over the kingdom. But not David. He spent the next couple of decades running from the current king, Saul, and refusing to take advantage of the opportunities he had to kill "the LORD's anointed" (1 Samuel 24:6; 26:8-11).

So what's the lesson for people struggling with infertility? It's quite simple. Although some people claim that God told them they were going to have a baby, most of us have received no such promise. I've had people tell me they were sure I was going to get pregnant, but I never got a personal message from God telling me to start getting the nursery ready. At any rate, if David, who had it from a very reliable source that he was going to be the next king, was willing to wait for God's timing, how much more should we, who have received no such guarantee that we are *ever* going to get pregnant, be willing to do the same?

This brings up a rather confusing question. When is it okay to pursue medical treatment, and when does such a pursuit become a sinful attempt to have our own way? I found my answer to that dilemma in a principle that Henry Blackaby and Claude King introduce in their well-known study *Experiencing God*.

The authors base their study about knowing and doing the will of God on seven key principles. Two of them—"God is always at work around you," and "God invites you to become involved with Him in His work"—were particularly meaningful to me as I was contemplating various infertility treatment options, particularly IVF.

These truths imply that we have two choices in life. Either we can start something and hope that God will join us in it (which tends to create fear, worry, anxiety, etc.)—or we can join Him in what He's already doing (which brings joy, peace, and contentment). As I thought about this, I concluded that for me, doing in vitro (or any other procedure that involved manipulating eggs and sperm outside the womb) would be akin to starting something and expecting God to join me. I didn't want to do that. So my only option was to cross IVF off my list of potential infertility solutions.

Don't get me wrong. I believe that God causes conception to occur, no matter where it takes place. And just because people try to start the process on their own doesn't mean that God is not involved in or in control of it. But based on testimonies I've read and heard, I also think that sometimes He allows people to get pregnant through various ARTs even though He might have had greater blessings in store for them had they just been willing to trust Him—and not been so anxious to make a pregnancy happen.

You may come to a different conclusion about IVF and other ARTs, and that's fine. What I've written is my own personal conviction, not a hard-and-fast rule for everyone. My opinion about

IVF really isn't your primary concern, anyway. At this point, your focus should be on trying to determine what, if anything, God wants *you* to do regarding the medical treatment of your infertility. Based on what I have learned, however, I do have one suggestion. After you evaluate each option from a financial, physical, personal, relational, and ethical perspective, submit it to the "joining God" test. Ask yourself, "By doing this, am I starting something and expecting God to join me?" An affirmative answer is a pretty clear indication that, if you do what you're considering, you'll be attempting to break down a door that probably should remain closed for now.

The Peace Filter

I hope the questions I've asked and the thought processes I've shared in the last two chapters will guide you as you evaluate the forms of medical intervention that might help you conceive. No matter how you approach this process, one thing is certain: There are no quick and easy answers. There definitely are certain moral and ethical boundaries that people who believe in the sanctity of human life are obligated not to cross. However, there is no one-size-fits-all formula for deciding what's acceptable and what's not when it comes to infertility treatment.

It's not my job to judge you for anything you may choose to do in your quest to get pregnant. Ultimately, those decisions are between you and God. And fortunately, He doesn't dangle choices in front of you and expect you to automatically know what to do. The Bible doesn't mention IVF, GIFT, ZIFT, or any other high-tech infertility procedure, but it certainly provides plenty of filters through which decisions about such ARTs can be made.

Will doing the procedure or treatment enhance your relationships with others, including your spouse? Will it foster love and unity—or will it create jealousy, bitterness, or dissension in your home? Does it show respect for human life? Is it a good use of the financial resources God has given you? Are your motives for pursuing this treatment pure, or are you doing it out of selfish ambition? Do you want to do it because you believe it's God will for your life, or because you are tired of waiting for Him to answer your prayers for a baby? Will it ultimately bring glory to God or to man?

If the procedure you're contemplating passes through these and other biblical filters, you have only one more question to ask yourself: Do you have peace about it?

Your focus should be on trying to determine what, if anything, God wants you to do regarding the medical treatment of your infertility.

If you have committed your infertility treatment to God every step along the way, and if you've been consistently asking for His will to be done as opposed to your own, the peace of God will be the tool that enables you to make the right decision, no matter what the issue.

The apostle Paul stressed the importance of this in Colossians 3:15 when he encouraged believers to "let the peace of God rule in your hearts" (NKJV). In this verse, the word "rule" means "'to serve as an arbiter,' or to use a contemporary term, 'to act as an umpire.'"[4] An umpire calls the shots—he is the final authority when questions or disputes arise in a game. This is the role that the peace of God plays in the hearts of believers. When you're trying to make a final decision about something, the presence of God's peace is a green light, and the absence of God's peace is a red light.

Let's say you're feeling very calm and settled after thoroughly evaluating IVF and deciding upon the limits you would want to place on the procedure. Is it okay for you to proceed? I see no reason why not. On the flip side, maybe you've examined intrauterine insemination from every possible angle and come to the conclusion that it is morally acceptable—but you still have an uneasy feeling about it. Should you do it? No.

You know how you feel when you're not experiencing peace. You need to pay attention to those feelings. When Randy and I were making decisions about infertility treatment, we followed a simple rule of thumb: When in doubt, don't. For us, feelings of doubt signified a lack of peace, and we weren't about to do anything if we didn't have complete peace about it first.

It was a lack of peace that made us decide to stop seeing the reproductive endocrinologist who had performed my surgeries. We just didn't feel right about pursuing treatment with him. In fact, as I mentioned in the chapter on God sightings, I was ready to stop trying to conceive altogether before we switched to the local gynecologist I now see.

Ironically, while we were unsettled about seeking further treatment with the specialist, we did have peace about doing some of the same procedures later. Sometimes, a lack of peace about a certain course of action may be tied to a specific set of circumstances. Once those circumstances change, the peace returns and we are free to proceed. In my case, for example, I believe the uneasy feeling I had about going through artificial insemination at the specialist's clinic was the tool God used to direct us to a doctor we were much more comfortable with.

The details of your situation may be different from mine. In fact, they probably are. But the overriding principle applies to all of us, no matter who we are or how long we've been dealing with infertility. When we commit our steps to God, He sends His peace to guard our hearts, protect our minds, and keep us from making decisions that we might regret later.

No Regrets

When your heart is aching to hold a baby of your own, it's difficult to think into the future much further than a month or two at a time. With infertility treatment, however, you're making decisions that you'll have to live with for the rest of your life, so you have a great responsibility to consider your options very carefully.

Randy and I took this responsibility seriously. We made our decisions together, and we consciously relinquished our right to second-guess ourselves later. When we decided not to pursue IVF, for example, we said to each other, "This is our choice, and we are not going to look back at it in ten years and wish we had done it differently."

As a result, we can honestly say that we have no regrets about the decisions we made. We can look back and know that we did everything we were willing to do. We didn't get the results we had hoped for, but we do have peace, and I wouldn't trade that for all the biological babies in the world.

TEN

While You Wait

❦

*I*n the early years of my marriage, I worked as a newspaper reporter covering business news in northwest Arkansas, home to such industry leaders as Wal-Mart Stores, Tyson Foods, and J.B. Hunt Transport Services. It had never been my goal to be a reporter. In fact, though I majored in journalism in college, the thought of working for a newspaper scared me to death. But jobs in public relations—which is what I thought I wanted—were hard to come by when I moved to that area of Arkansas. That's how I ended up with a reporter's notebook in my hand.

I began my career at a small local newspaper. Eventually I went to work for the *Arkansas Democrat-Gazette*, the statewide paper. Although I liked some aspects of the job—meeting entrepreneurial people, researching interesting topics, and feeling good about well-written articles—I looked forward to the day when I could quit and stay at home with my first child.

By the time Randy and I started trying to get pregnant, my job had become quite stressful, and I began to view having a baby as my way out. I would work until the seventh or eighth month of my pregnancy, I decided, and then spend those last several weeks preparing my heart and home for motherhood.

There was only one problem. Even as I was making these plans, I was beginning to realize that conception wasn't going to be as easy as I had hoped. To make matters worse, as month after month went by without a missed period, I was becoming increasingly frustrated at work. The aspects of my job that I had enjoyed were no longer fun, and an overzealous editor was driving me crazy.

These two factors—no pregnancy and a growing dissatisfaction with my job—were a bad combination. This was especially so because in my mind, the former was going to save me from the latter. I was planning my future around something I wasn't even sure was going to occur, and as a result, I became stuck on a never-ending merry-go-round of anxiety, stress, and discontentment.

It's easy to fall into this kind of trap when you're trying to get pregnant. You have a specific goal in mind, and it seems as if everything in your life is either oriented toward achieving that goal or contingent upon the realization of that goal. Phrases such as "When I get pregnant..." and "When we have a baby..." no longer trigger an occasional daydream—they become the main focus of nearly all your thoughts and conversations.

There's nothing wrong with looking forward to having a child—it's a normal and healthy part of marriage. When infertility is thrown into the mix, however, life can get out of balance very quickly. Attempting to get pregnant can be like a full-time job. Everything you do, from intimate activity with your spouse to the scheduling of vacations, is governed by your ovulation schedule and accompanying visits to the doctor's office for this test or that procedure. You're always waiting for something—a blood test, a shot, a prescription, a meeting with the infertility specialist, a phone call from the nurse, an ultrasound, another blood test, the day your period will start if you're not pregnant, and so on.

When so much of your physical and emotional energy is devoted to trying to conceive, it's often difficult to function, let alone to try to be joyful and fulfilled. But life must go on, even when you're waiting for a positive pregnancy test. Otherwise, you'll wake up one day and realize the sad truth that you spent the past three, five, or seven years living solely for the future. And perhaps you'll have nothing to show for it.

Fortunately, there are plenty of things that you can do (or not do, as the case may be) to make the wait for a baby bearable, and maybe even productive. Although infertility is an unwelcome intrusion that requires a great deal of time and attention, you can make it easier on yourself and your emotions by wisely managing the aspects of life over which you do have some control.

Just Say No

One of the best things you can do for yourself while you're battling infertility is to develop a higher level of emotional intelligence about your situation. That might sound intimidating, but it's really not. It simply involves becoming more aware of how you react in various situations. Then you use those reactions to help you determine what you can and cannot handle when it comes to baby showers, Mother's Day services at church, and even strolls through the infant department at your local department store.

Let's say practically everyone you know is having a baby, and you're being inundated with shower invitations. You love your friends, and you want to share in their joy, but every time you go to Babies "R" Us to buy another shower gift, you end up in tears for the rest of the day. Going to the actual shower is even worse. That usually sets you back emotionally for at least an entire day, sometimes two. Here's where a little emotional intelligence comes in handy. If you know that baby showers really bother you, don't go. Just send your friend a card and a nice gift certificate a few days before the party, and then on the day of the event, stay home and rent a good chick flick instead. If the mother-to-be is a good enough friend to invite you to her baby shower, she ought to understand why you can't attend. And if she doesn't, don't worry about it. You need to do what's best for you and your emotional well-being.

The same applies to Mother's Day services and baby dedications at church, social gatherings where you know there will be hordes of infants and toddlers running around, family-oriented

Attempting to get pregnant can be like a full-time job.

events such as holiday fireworks displays and church picnics, and window-shopping at stores that specialize in baby or maternity clothing. If such activities simply serve as excruciating reminders of the painful fact that you don't have any children, it may be advisable to avoid them. Obviously, you won't be able to steer clear of every situation like this. However, if you have a choice about the matter, don't put yourself into positions where you know you're going to get upset. Just say no.

To keep from having to wipe your social calendar completely clean, pay attention to how you respond to various situations at different times of the month. You might find that you are able to shop for baby gifts, attend showers, or enjoy children's choir programs at church during the first half of your cycle, while you're better off staying home if the dates of such events fall closer to the start of your period.

The better you know yourself, the more skilled you will be at avoiding situations and events that are hazardous to your emotional health. This reminds me of a joke I heard years ago that went something like this:

Patient: "Doctor, I broke my arm in three places."

Doctor: "Stay outta them places."

When you're dealing with infertility, there are times when you need to use this doctor's commonsense approach and stay away from the places that cause you pain. You might miss out on some fun. You'll probably disappoint a few friends. But your heart will thank you for it later.

A Relational Safety Net

Another tricky aspect of infertility is figuring out how to cope with the fact that your friends—at least the ones around your age who have been married about as long as you—all seem to be having babies while you remain childless. The void in your life is particularly obvious when you get together for coffee, lunch, or "just to talk." After a while, listening to your girlfriends discuss diaper rash, formula, nursing, and a zillion other similar topics gets really old, especially since you don't have anything to contribute to the conversation.

Other women who are also having trouble getting pregnant can provide some welcome relief from all the baby talk. And few things are more comforting than sharing your struggles with a close friend who is going through the same trial. But there's always the chance that these women will get pregnant too. As bad as it sounds, trying to be happy for a former infertility patient can be even more difficult than rejoicing when a very fertile friend has another baby. (Misery loves company, remember?)

So are infertile women doomed to lives of friendless loneliness? I don't think so. The answer to this dilemma lies in forming close relationships with Christian friends who are in a totally different season of life. You don't have to turn your back on all your friends with toddlers, of course. But if you have the opportunity to get to know some older women with teenage or young adult children, or perhaps no children at all, by all means do it. I have been blessed to have a few such friends in my life, and I would be hard-pressed to tell you how much their prayers and encouragement have meant to me during the last few years.

These friends are "safe." I don't have to worry about them surprising me with the news that they are pregnant. Most of them never had fertility problems, but they've all been through other life-changing trials that stretched and refined their faith. They may not know what it's like to experience infertility firsthand, but they do know what it's like to experience God's apparent silence and wonder what He's up to in their lives. I've been strengthened and inspired by their wisdom, their compassion, and their godly examples.

If you don't know any women who could fill this relational void in your life, you might be able to meet some by getting involved in a ladies' Bible study or some type of community outreach ministry at your church. And don't forget to pray about it. God knows how important friends are. In His time, He'll bring someone into your life who will encourage you in your faith and help you bear the heavy burden of infertility.

Rose-Colored Glasses

The longer your desire to become a parent goes unfulfilled, the easier it is to start idealizing motherhood and looking at having children through rose-colored glasses. You long for a newborn baby to kiss and cuddle. You ache for tiny hands to hold and soft skin to rub. So you begin to picture an idyllic life in which your perfect little angel loves to play quietly and take long naps, learns to walk by the time she's eight months old, is potty trained at 16 months, and always gets along famously with all her preschool friends.

That *could* happen, I suppose, but reality is usually a bit more challenging. Babies are a ton of work. They cry—a lot. They wake you up at all hours of the night. They get sick. They spit up. They eat things they were never intended to eat. They disobey. They require constant attention.

But that's only the beginning. As much as you'd like them to stay cute and cuddly forever, they eventually become teenagers. And then the fun really starts. They rebel. They get hurt. They fight with their siblings—and with you. They get acne. They experience rejection. They make mistakes, sometimes really big ones.

Most books for prospective or expectant parents say nothing about the job of a parent once those precious little bundles of joy grow up. They don't explain how to teach children right from wrong, or how to handle money wisely, or how to resist temptation. They don't mention that someday, your job description may include comforting a child whose best friend was killed in a car accident, helping your son deal with bullies at school, or (God forbid) working through the trauma of sexual molestation with your daughter.

I'm not suggesting that the joys of being a parent don't significantly outweigh the pain. Or that people should elect not to have children so they don't have to deal with any of this. I do believe, however, that remembering the more difficult aspects of parenting can help you maintain a healthy attitude while you're trying to conceive. Viewing motherhood through rose-colored glasses will not make the wait any easier. It will only make you less content and more miserable.

This is another reason why it's good to have friends with teenage or young adult children. Listening to them discuss their older children's struggles and problems will give you a good dose of reality about what parenting is all about. And perhaps it will keep you from viewing having a baby as a cure-all for your problems and worries.

A Chance of Showers

As part of a "get-to-know-each-other" exercise in a class at church, I once had to describe my personality as a weather report. I mulled it over for a few minutes and decided that words such as "calm" and "cool" best summed me up. After hearing my assessment, Randy added one more element to my personality forecast: It also included a chance of showers, he said.

The more I thought about that, the more I realized that his description painted a pretty accurate picture of my emotional state when we were trying to conceive. I wasn't angry or bitter or despondent all the time. There was always a slight chance of showers in my world, though. There was always the possibility that something—anything—would cause my eyes to fill with tears and a lump to form in my throat. Dealing with the onslaught of emotions that accompanies infertility was very frustrating for me. I was constantly trying to figure out why I was crying about this and why I was feeling sad about that. And when I wasn't attempting to figure all that out, I was trying to talk myself out of feeling bad in the first place.

I eventually realized that I didn't have to explain away my emotions. I understood that it's perfectly natural to feel depressed or numb for awhile, to cry for no apparent reason, and to go through phases where all I wanted to do was curl up into a little ball under my bed and stay there for a week. Such feelings didn't mean that I needed to be committed to a mental hospital (although I'm sure the thought did occur to Randy once or twice). Neither did they indicate that I was responding in a sinful or unspiritual manner. They simply showed that I was a normal human being who was grieving because my God-given desire to reproduce and nurture was being hampered by physical problems that were out of my control.

If your emotional struggles with infertility are interfering with your ability to handle daily life—if you're experiencing depression that doesn't lift, high levels of anxiety, persistent feelings of bitterness or anger, or thoughts about suicide or death, for example—you might consider seeking help from a professional Christian counselor. There's nothing wrong with receiving outside assistance. Some trials are just too difficult to handle alone. And for some people, infertility is one of them.

Thankfully, most people survive the emotional ups and downs of infertility, with or without professional help. Some, of course, are a little worse for the wear. But they eventually realize that the sun *will* come out tomorrow, even if the storm is raging furiously around them today. As the psalmist wrote, "Weeping may endure for a night, but joy comes in the morning" (Psalm 30:5, NKJV).

Combating the Sadness

That said, there are some things you can do to ward off or neutralize the bouts of sadness or depression you'll likely experience as you're waiting for morning to come. For example, exercise is one of the most effective antidepressants I've discovered so far. That may be the last thing you want to hear right now, but it really does work. The endorphins that the brain releases during intense physical activity have been proven to lighten moods and make people feel better. If I wake up in the morning feeling somewhat depressed or blue, a half hour on the treadmill is usually all it takes to cheer me up a bit. You may prefer walking or running outside, swimming, aerobics or some other kind of exercise. It doesn't matter what you do, as long as you're doing something. (Come to think of it, what better time to get into shape than when you're trying to conceive? If you get pregnant, you'll be much better equipped to carry the baby—and if you don't, you'll still look and feel better, which will help you combat feelings of inadequacy you may have because of your infertility.)

Creative activities such as gardening, woodworking, scrap-booking, silk-flower arranging, and sewing also can combat mood swings and help make the wait for a baby a bit easier. You may not know how to do any of these things, but again, there's no time like the present to learn. Before I started trying to get pregnant, I didn't know the first thing about gardening. Since then, I've gotten so hooked that I recently took a master-gardener class through my county's cooperative extension service. There's just something about digging around in my flowerbeds, yanking weeds out of the ground, and watching plants grow and change that makes me forget all that's wrong in the world.

It may sound a bit odd, but gardening also has helped me develop my nurturing side. My flowers and houseplants obviously

The better you know yourself, the more skilled you will be at avoiding situations and events that are hazardous to your emotional health.

can't take the place of a baby in my life, but they are alive, and they do respond when I give them proper care. My point is this: If you've always wanted to learn how to garden, paint, arrange flowers, sew, or take professional-looking photographs, don't put it off any longer. Sign up for a night class at your local community college or technical institute. It might be just what the doctor ordered to cure your waiting-for-baby blues.

If you want to prevent some emotional lows, I'd encourage you to refrain from purchasing anything baby-related until you have a positive pregnancy test. You might be tempted to buy a maternity dress or two, some cute little baby outfits, a mobile for the crib, or any number of other accessories for the nursery. But seeing such items will only make you feel worse about the fact that you're having trouble conceiving. Of course you want to participate in all the joy and excitement that other prospective parents get to experience. But this is one area where it really is better to practice a little discipline.

If you already have some baby things, put them all in a box and stick the box in a closet where you don't have to look at it. You already have to deal with plenty of reminders that you're not pregnant—there's no need to suffer additional heartache if you can avoid it.

Praying for God's will to be done regarding your family (see chapter four for a recap) also can help control or alleviate the emotional turmoil that often comes with the onset of yet another period. Some people spend hours or even days crying each month. The devastation is even more acute when the lack of a pregnancy means that a costly infertility procedure didn't work. Because of my physical condition, I usually had a pretty good idea that my period was on its way a few days before it actually started. This could have been why I never experienced such utter despair when that time of the month rolled around again. But I truly believe it was praying for God's will to be done in my life that eased my sorrow the most and kept me from having an emotional earthquake every month.

I knew that if I wasn't pregnant, it wasn't because Randy and I hadn't timed things right. It wasn't because the doctor had made a mistake when he did the IUI. It was because God had kept my womb closed yet again. I was terribly disappointed each time that happened, of course. But I was also comforted by the fact that, even though I didn't understand it, this was all part of God's mysterious plan for my life. He didn't turn His back on me when I was hurting, but He didn't let my tears change His mind about what He had in store for me, either. And somehow—only by His infinite mercy and grace, I'm sure—I was okay with that.

It's Not All About You

Infertility is a difficult trial. There's no doubt about it. It's overwhelming, it's frustrating, it's confusing, and it's painful. As a result, it's very easy to become so consumed by it that you start acting like the whole world revolves around you and your inability to get pregnant. This tendency isn't exclusive to infertility, of course. It can happen with any hardship, from marital crises and financial problems to workplace dilemmas and terminal illnesses. But the fact that it's not limited to people who are struggling to conceive doesn't mean that it's an acceptable way to live.

When you're waiting for a baby, one of the biggest challenges you face is the danger of become too self-absorbed. You can start viewing every conversation and every offhand remark as a direct assault on you and your infertility. If you're with a group of parents and they start asking each other what they ever talked about before they had children, you think they're implying that your life is meaningless and empty because you and your spouse don't have children. If a pastor or Sunday school teacher mentions that he considers his children to be among the greatest blessings in his life, you bristle because you're sure what he really means is that your life is cursed because you don't have any children. If your friends fail to ask you how you're handling your infertility every time they see you, you take offense at their obvious lack of care and concern for you. And on it goes.

These people really might be insensitive clods like those we talked about in chapter seven. But most of the time, their comments have absolutely nothing to do with you and your inability to get pregnant. When new parents wonder what they talked about before they had kids, they're not making a judgment about you and your life. Rather, they're just marveling about the huge change that has recently occurred in their own lives. Sure, it would be nice if they were a bit more sensitive when you're around. However, the truth of the matter is that (unlike you, perhaps) they simply aren't thinking about your infertility every waking minute.

As much as we'd like everyone on earth to be aware of our pain, the fact is that most people have no reason to think about infertility. We are only setting ourselves up for disappointment when we expect them to know about it. In addition, as we learned in chapter six, just because other people have what we want (namely, children) does not necessarily mean that their lives are perfect. Every person has his or her own set of problems, challenges, and issues. And most are so engrossed in handling their own lives that they don't have time to think negative thoughts about ours.

I'm stressing this so emphatically because I've fallen prey to the self-absorption trap myself (on more than one occasion). I can assure you that all it does is make infertility even more of a mental and emotional battle. When you're constantly interpreting what other people say from the perspective of someone who can't have children, you tend to get offended quite easily. And who wants to run around feeling insulted all the time? On top of that, you can be so busy getting your feelings hurt that you can miss out on the obvious humor and irony in another person's story. (And God knows you can always use a little laughter when you're waiting for a baby!)

I was reminded of this several weeks ago as I was listening to a friend talk about her daughter-in-law. She had found out she was pregnant a few days *after* her husband had gotten a vasectomy. The couple already had three children and apparently had decided that was enough. Judging by the surprise pregnancy, however, God had other plans. As I sat there listening to the other women around me express surprise and amazement about this situation, I experienced a strange mixture of emotions. On one hand, the irony of the situation certainly wasn't lost on me. I could relate to the daughter-in-law's shock at making this discovery after having taken such a drastic step to prevent it from happening. But I also had a tiny twinge of irritability at the thought that a woman was upset (at least initially) because she was pregnant.

As I mulled this over later, I realized once again that the sun does not rise and set around my infertility. I would love to become pregnant unexpectedly. But I can see how that kind of surprise would turn the worlds of many married couples completely upside-down. Rather than get all worked up about the inequity of the situation (that would only have made me miserable), I chose to view it for what it was: an interesting story about a surprising turn of events.

As hard as infertility is, it's not all there is to life. So the next time your inability to conceive starts wearing you down, force yourself to look around and start viewing the world from someone else's perspective. What you discover might make you laugh. It might make you cry. And it might even help you realize you're not the only one in the world with problems.

Comfort Experience

This realization often opens the door to ministry opportunities that you may have never known existed. In fact, you probably weren't prepared to handle them before your battle with infertility.

Let me explain what I mean. When I was struggling to conceive and dealing with the medical problems caused by my endometriosis, I often wondered what this trial was preparing me for. I had it in my head that God was getting me ready for some *really* horrible ordeal—that my infertility was some kind of training course for whatever awful thing was going to happen to me in the future.

I have no idea what lies around the next bend in the road, much less what's going to happen in a few years or more. For all I know, it may very well be something terrible. But rather than dwell on that possibility, I eventually came to view my struggles with infertility in a different light. Rather than thinking of what Randy and I were going through as some kind of boot camp for future suffering, I started to think of it as an opportunity to gain what I like to call "comfort experience."

The more my heart hurt over my inability to conceive, the more aware I became of other people's pain. I began to understand that, although the trappings may be different, the effects of pain

> *He didn't turn His back on me when I was hurting, but He didn't let my tears change His mind about what He had in store for me, either. And somehow—only by His infinite mercy and grace, I'm sure—I was okay with that.*

are universal. It doesn't matter if the suffering is due to an unfaithful spouse, cancer, strained family relationships, a failed business deal, wayward children, a tragic accident, or the death of a parent. It's still suffering. It still makes people wander around in circles in their kitchens (or garages or living rooms), numbly wondering how they are going to make it through another day, much less another month or year. It still makes them cry themselves to sleep at night, completely exhausted from praying prayers that seem to fall on deaf ears.

As I waited for some kind of resolution to my infertility, I learned what it meant to feel the pain of others. I had never been very empathetic. In fact, I was probably guilty of "comforting" people by rattling off pat spiritual answers more times than I care to remember. But being on the receiving end of such "encouragement" made me realize just how empty and ineffective it really is. It taught me that people who are suffering don't want answers—they just want to know that someone cares about them and understands that they're hurting.

I didn't become a master comforter overnight. But gradually, as I began to pay more attention to what was going on around me, I started to notice more situations in which I could offer a compassionate word or lend a sympathetic ear. These opportunities weren't forced. They happened because my own suffering had made me more attentive to the needs of others. The apostle Paul summed up this process in 2 Corinthians 1:3-4: "Praise be to the God and Father of our Lord Jesus Christ, the Father of compassion and the God of all comfort, who comforts us in all our troubles, *so that we can comfort those in any trouble with the comfort we ourselves have received from God.*"

If you do nothing else while you're waiting for a baby, use your struggles with infertility as an opportunity to gain comfort experience. Watch how other people react to individuals who are suffering. Use what you see—both the positive and the negative—to improve the way you respond in similar situations.

Above all else, learn to listen. It's natural to want to tell your stories and share your experiences, but hurting people don't need to hear about someone else's pain. They need someone who will listen to *them*. And with your newfound (perhaps) empathy skills, you might be just the person for the job.

A Calling

Many people, including many Christians, view infertility as an obstacle they have to overcome so they can get on with the rest of their lives. They fail to consider the possibility that their inability to conceive is not an accident—that if they are childless, it's because God ordained for them to be so, at least temporarily. We covered all this back in the first few chapters. But as we talk about what to do while you wait for a baby, I want to remind you of one very important truth.

In God's schedule of events for your life, infertility is not some in-between phase you just have to get through before you can get on with your "real" life. It's a calling.

Yes, you read that right. If you have not been able to conceive, then at this point in your life, God has called you to be infertile. I'm not saying the calling is permanent. Neither am I saying that you are required to enjoy it. But I am saying that God knows what He's doing, and if He isn't allowing you to become pregnant right now, it is because He has some other purpose to fulfill.

When you view infertility as a calling, rather than as a barrier in the road or a crimp in your plans, you're much more likely to experience peace and joy in the midst of your sorrow. And you have a much greater chance of actually discovering what God wants you to do during this season of life. Because whether you want to believe it or not, God *does* have a job for you to do while you're waiting for a baby. Ephesians 2:10 makes this clear: "We are God's workmanship, created in Christ Jesus to do good works, which God prepared in advance for us to do."

On the other hand, you can allow your life to become a continual waiting game. But then you run the risk of missing the assignments that God has planned for you today—assignments that have the potential to bless your life in ways you can't even imagine. Don't be so consumed by your plans to conceive a baby and have a perfect little family that you forget your life right now. You can plan for the future—but don't *live* for the future.

That's exactly what I was doing when I was working at the newspaper. For a time, my whole life was focused on one goal—getting pregnant so I could quit. Eventually, however, I decided that I couldn't base my career decisions on whether or not I had a baby. I left the newspaper, even though I wasn't pregnant and didn't have another job (or any serious prospects of getting one—at least not immediately).

Taking "early retirement" from the newspaper business was one of the best moves I ever made. The stress in my life decreased exponentially. I began to explore other interests and develop skills I never knew I possessed. And life around the Flowers home became much, much happier.

Looking back, I'm very glad I had godly people in my life who counseled me to make that change when I did. If I had stuck to my original plan of not quitting until I was seven months pregnant, I'd still be there, plugging away at a job I didn't like, continually stressed out over things that didn't really matter, and perpetually miserable because my dream of becoming a mother wasn't coming true.

John Lennon once wisely observed, "Life is what happens when you're busy making other plans." When you're waiting for a baby, it's easy to let the joys and blessings of life pass you by because you're so intent on achieving your goal of growing your family.

Don't let that happen to you. Don't miss out on an abundant life today because you're so engrossed in making plans for tomorrow. Life really is too short for that.

ELEVEN

Letting Go of the Dream

❦

*B*efore I got married, a dear friend gave me a tiny hand-knit sweater that she had lovingly crafted out of powder-blue yarn. With its intricate stitching and cute little baseball buttons, it was the perfect gift for a young bride-to-be who was full of dreams about the baby boy she hoped to have one day.

For many years, I kept that sweater in my hope chest, nestled in the same tissue paper it was in when my friend gave it to me. It was, of course, waiting for the arrival of our first son. I knew he would look especially adorable in it, particularly if he inherited his father's blue eyes and mischievous smile.

The sweater is still in the hope chest, but it's no longer as visible or accessible as it once was. Several months ago, as I was wrapping Christmas presents for my family, I put it in a box so I would no longer have to look at it every time I opened the lid of the hope chest.

This might seem like a rather minor move—a simple matter of rearranging a storage space. But for me, it was a significant turning point.

As I had thought about what to give my pregnant older sister, I had gone to the hope chest and pulled the sweater out of its tissue wrapping. I didn't know whether she was having a boy or a girl, so I didn't know if such a present would even be appropriate. I just knew I wanted to give her something special—a gift to help her celebrate the fact that after two heartbreaking miscarriages, it appeared that she was finally going to realize *her* dream of becoming a mother.

Tears filled my eyes as I thought about what this little garment signified. For so long, I had dreamed of the day when I would place it on my newborn son as we got ready to bring him home from the hospital. I could picture the three of us on our way home—a proud daddy, a tired-but-happy mommy, and a chubby little cherub all decked out in his brand new sweater.

Back then, the sweater was a symbol of bright hope, a precious indicator of wonderful things to come. Years later, however, it was a bittersweet reminder of what will probably never be. If we continue to build our family through international adoption, any babies we bring home in the future will likely be too big for the little blue sweater. I really had no reason to keep it.

And yet I still have it. I didn't give it to my sister—I put it in a gift box and stuck it back in the hope chest. I'm not sure why I decided to keep it, aside from the fact that Randy encouraged me not to give it away. It was made for me and my baby, he said, and it wouldn't be right for anyone else to have it.

More than half a year later, I'm glad I followed his advice. Instead of reminding me of what I don't have, the sweater now represents the release of a dream. You see, by the time the clenched fingers of my heart relaxed enough to let that dream go, an even more wonderful reality was waiting to take its place. It wasn't necessarily the reality we would have chosen if we had been given a say in the matter. But it was the reality that God had chosen for us. And the sooner we accepted it, the easier it would be to joyfully embark on the next chapter in our lives.

Thinking About Release

I realize that when you have your heart set on getting pregnant and giving birth to a beautiful, healthy child, the last thing you want to think about is the possibility that your vision for your family might not play out the way you had hoped. But there's always a chance that it won't. In mid-2002, RESOLVE, a national organization for infertile couples, stated on its Web site that "roughly two-thirds of couples who seek medical intervention [for infertility] are able to give birth."[1] The unstated corollary, of course, is that about 33 percent of couples do *not* respond to treatment with a successful pregnancy.

I don't want to be the bearer of bad news, but that 33 percent *could* include you. I hope it doesn't, but it might. And if it does, there will come a day in your life when you, too, will have to let your dream of a biological child go.

You don't just wake up one morning and decide that you're over your infertility. It would be nice if it worked that way, but it doesn't. Designating a specific stopping point and ceasing treatment when that point comes is an important first step. It's only the beginning, though. Letting go of the dream to conceive is a gradual process, one that involves a significant amount of grief and loss. But despite the pain involved, it must be done. Otherwise, you will never be able to embrace whatever "alternate" plan God is already unfolding for your life.

I can't tell you how many months or years you should devote to infertility treatment—that's for you and your spouse to decide. But I can tell you that it is okay to quit. As un-American as it sounds, it's okay to give up. Although your friends and family may suggest otherwise, closing the door on further efforts to get pregnant doesn't signify a lack of faith. It doesn't mean that you are weak or unspiritual. It doesn't imply that you really didn't want a baby in the first place. It simply means that you recognize that "there is a time for everything, and a season for every activity under heaven," including "a time to search [for conception, in this case] and a time to give up" (Ecclesiastes 3:1,6).

Some people are so intent on achieving a pregnancy that they have difficulty acknowledging this truth. Even after six miscarriages, or seven failed in vitro attempts, or a dozen artificial inseminations, or ten years of carefully timed intercourse, they're still holding out hope that a successful pregnancy remains within their grasp.

I'm not saying this couldn't happen—we've all heard stories about people who conceived after 15 years of trying or those who finally gave birth after losing numerous pregnancies. But there

You don't just wake up one morning and decide that you're over your infertility.

comes a time when every couple must evaluate the emotional, physical, and financial consequences of further treatment and utter these three little words: "Enough is enough." If the wife is unwilling or unable to call it quits, the husband must step up and do it. In his God-given role as protector of his family, he is responsible for the emotional, physical, and spiritual health of his wife. And it doesn't take a doctorate in psychology to figure out that numerous miscarriages or a decade of continual disappointment can do irreversible damage to a person's heart and soul.

I don't know where you are in your personal journey. But I have a feeling that if you've made it this far in this book, you have a pretty good idea whether you need to pay particularly close attention to what I'm about to say. I'm not suggesting that those of you who are in the earlier stages of infertility can skip this part. Any reading you can do now that may help you cope later is worth the time and effort, as far as I'm concerned. But I'm writing this chapter especially for those of you who are tired of fighting a losing battle with infertility, as well as for those of you who have already given up trying to get pregnant but are still trying to accept the reality that you'll never have biological children.

It's difficult to admit that it might be time to stop. It's also tough to let go of a hurt that has been festering for many years. Neither process is without pain—in fact, you're probably going to feel worse before you feel better. That's the way healing is. But unlike human doctors who make mistakes and can't always make people well, our Great Physician never misdiagnoses anything, and He can heal the most serious of conditions—a broken heart.

As you read this chapter, you may need to stop every now and then and cry out to Him for courage and strength to keep going. I've already had to do that, and I've only written a few paragraphs. Thankfully, as we learned in chapter two, "The LORD is close to the brokenhearted and saves those who are crushed in spirit" (Psalm 34:18). He's always close by, ready to comfort you and give you fresh hope for tomorrow.

Let the Rains Begin

You're going to need that comforting touch, especially when you start to deal with all the things you will never get to experience. Acknowledging these desires might be almost more than you can bear, but it's an important step toward acceptance. Make a list of all those events and milestones that you have looked forward to for so long, along with the feeling you expected to experience with each one. Then, one by one, release them to God in prayer.

I'll get you started with some items from my own list:

- The joy of a positive pregnancy test.

- The anxiety of waiting out those first few months with high hopes of carrying the child to full term.
- The thrill of telling friends and family—many of whom have been praying and hoping with you for years—that "we're pregnant."
- The anticipation of finding out whether you're going to have a boy or a girl.
- The honor of giving your parents their first grandchild (or, as I hoped to do, the first granddaughter in the family).
- The excitement of registering for infant gifts.
- The fun of packing your bag for the hospital.
- The nervousness of waiting for your water to break.
- The exhilaration of making it through labor and holding your newborn for the very first time.

This assignment is draining. But it's only the tip of the iceberg when it comes to the emotional upheaval you will likely experience as you move closer to relinquishing your dream of conceiving. Unfortunately, the monthly emotional roller coaster you rode when you were trying to get pregnant doesn't stop when you call it quits. It keeps going. Only instead of being on a monthly schedule, it becomes much more random.

Remember how Randy said that my personality included a "chance of showers"? This is a case in point. Even now, I can't always predict what is going to trigger the rain. Tears often come at the most inopportune times. They might start when I'm driving down the road and a song that was especially meaningful to me at some point in my infertility journey comes on the radio. They may well up when a commercial on television reminds me that I'll probably never have a reason to "think I may be pregnant." Or they may come when I'm talking to Randy—about some aspect of our past, our present, or even our future.

As I mentioned in the last chapter, I used to try to figure out the reason or the cause of these crying spells. I don't do that anymore. I simply view each one as another tiny step in the healing process. Crying is cathartic—like exercise, it causes the brain to release those wonderful endorphins that make us feel so much better. So don't resist the tears or view the inevitable downpours as a sign of weakness. They're not. As you grieve the losses that accompany infertility, don't be afraid to let the tears flow. Remember, "Those who sow in tears will reap with songs of joy" (Psalm 126:5).

Not the End of the World

Until now, I've purposely refrained from writing what I'm about to say because it's tough to digest, especially when the people around you are ambushing you with irritating advice and unhelpful encouragement. But it's time for some tough love. It's time for me to come right out and say that infertility is *not* the end of the world.

It's rough, I'll grant you that. It may be the most difficult thing you've ever had to face in your life. In the grand scheme of things, it might even rank up there with some of life's greatest inequities. But it's not the end of the world. People have died in childbirth and from dozens of other diseases and accidents. But I can't think of one woman who ever died because she couldn't have children. There *is* life after infertility, even though you might doubt it right now.

The world will keep turning. And if you're open to Plan B (which has actually been God's Plan A all along), you'll eventually be happy turning with it.

One way to accept this is to remember that you're not the only person who has ever had to give up a dream. I know, I know—if such a word of wisdom had come from someone with no experience with infertility, you'd have a right to be upset. I agree—that is definitely *not* a caring statement when it spills off the lips of a man or woman with three children. But take it from someone who knows. It can really help you keep your loss in perspective.

As I was struggling to conceive, I often forced myself to remember that people who have cancer and other terminal illnesses also have to give up their dreams. So do people who lose their businesses, their spouses (to death, desertion, or infidelity), or their innocence (due to rapists and molesters). Star athletes who get injured have to release dreams, as do accident victims who are confined to wheelchairs, families whose homes are consumed by fire, and children who lose their parents at an early age.

When you think about the agony associated with these tragedies, you start to realize that you are not alone in your suffering. You might even start to be just a little bit grateful that, of all the bad things that God could have allowed in your life, He chose to permit infertility.

The idea that other people have had to give up lifelong dreams was a huge comfort to me as I struggled to accept the fact that I couldn't have children. This notion may not be helpful to you right now, but as you make a conscious effort to take your eyes off yourself and your problems and turn them toward other people and their pain, I'm confident it will provide solace for you, too.

Painful Reminders

It also might come in handy after you've decided to stop trying to get pregnant, especially when you stumble across things that remind you of your infertility journey. You never know when you're going to happen upon these poignant "souvenirs." But trust me—it will happen.

I once had a huge infertility flashback when I was cleaning out the bottom of my microwave hutch. As I pulled out old vases, cookbooks, and containers of vitamins, I came across two small bottles—one partly filled with baby aspirin and the other with folic acid—both relics from my days of trying to get pregnant. As I looked at them, I recalled the doctor's orders: I was to take the baby aspirin because it might prevent miscarriage and the folic acid because of its potential to thwart certain birth defects.

Guess I didn't need those after all, I thought, strangely amused at the irony of the situation.

The pills brought back bittersweet memories. Although it would have been easy to stuff those recollections by tossing the bottles in the trash, my frugal nature wouldn't allow me to do that. Instead, I decided to take the folic acid—it's beneficial even for women who aren't pregnant—and I put the baby aspirin in our medicine drawer in case the daughter we are waiting to adopt ever needs them.

The discovery of these forgotten relics was somewhat emotional for me. I was surprised, though, to find that it wasn't a completely negative experience. It's not like I was cleaning out the dresser of a husband who had been killed in an airplane crash, or the closet of a child who had been run over by a drunk driver. The aspirin and the folic acid were reminders of a dream I had been forced to release. But the very fact that I was able to save the aspirin for my adopted child made me realize that, despite my loss, I still had much for which to be thankful.

Unfortunately, you won't be able to find the silver lining in all the clouds brought on by these reminders. With some, you just have to tell yourself that sometimes, life just isn't fair and you just have to make the best of it. That's what I had to do the last time I went to the doctor for my annual exam. I always dread going in for these regular visits. This particular year was no different. Although I was grateful that I didn't have to discuss any infertility issues with the doctor, I still wasn't looking forward to seeing all the pregnant women in the waiting room.

I purposely did not use the bathroom before I left the house because every other time I'd gone in for my annual exam, they had always taken a urine sample for a pregnancy test. Not this time, however. The nurse who took my vital signs didn't even ask me when my last period had started. *That* had never happened before. It was as if I had had a great big red "I" stamped on my chart—with the words "hopeless case" scrawled across it.

Talk about a massive dose of reality. I was barely 31 years old, and my childbearing years were apparently over. This was a sobering thought, even for someone who had mentally accepted that fact months earlier.

As I turned it over in my mind, I realized once again that infertility is something that never goes away completely. You might think you're totally okay with it. You might welcome several adopted children into your family with open arms. You might even feel called to turn your experiences into a book designed to help others in a similar situation. But you never really get over it.

Sure, the pain subsides, and other activities and pursuits occupy the time you once spent grieving the loss of your dream. But as much as you wish you could, you can never totally erase that scarlet "I" from the chart of your life. You might not introduce yourself to strangers by saying, "Hi, I'm Lois, and I can't have children," but infertility will forever remain a part of who you are.

As bleak as this sounds, it does *not* mean that you will be forever prevented from coming to spiritual closure regarding your inability to conceive. It might take you a while to work through all the theological questions that stem from your infertility. Eventually, though, you can become settled and at peace about this involuntary life assignment.

Accepting the "No"

For me, help with closure came from a rather unlikely source. I was in the shower one day, thinking about how the Bible says that Jesus can empathize with all our sorrows because He experienced every human emotion that we will ever experience (see Hebrews 2:18; 4:14-16). But Jesus wasn't a woman. So how could He possibly relate to the grief associated with not being able to conceive a baby? I know He never had biological children, so perhaps He could relate a little bit. But could He really understand?

That's when it hit me. I was focusing on the end result, not the process. Even though my infertility had a physical cause, my basic problem was a spiritual one: God had responded to my prayers with a resounding "no."

Therein lies my assurance that Jesus really did understand what I was going through. He wasn't a woman, so He didn't have my hormonal makeup, reproductive equipment, and maternal instinct. But at one point in His life—at the most pivotal cross-roads a human being could ever imagine—He too got a big fat "no" from God.

I've already used this example, but it bears repeating because the application is so relevant. When Jesus was in the garden of Gethsemane before His arrest and crucifixion, He asked God for another way *three times*. And all three times, God said no.

Think about the ramifications of God's answer. We're not talking about the disappointment of an unfulfilled dream here. We're talking about the inexpressible anguish of being separated from the presence of God after an eternity of togetherness. We're talking about the measureless agony of having your heavenly Father turn His back on you. We're talking about the excruciating pain of bearing the punishment for the sins of the world.

Does Jesus understand how it feels when God says no? Absolutely. Does He truly comprehend what it's like to experience the sorrow of infertility? Most definitely. He's not some comforter wannabe who would really like to empathize with you—but can't because He has two children and one on the way. As Isaiah 53:3 reveals, He's a "Man of sorrows and acquainted with grief" (NKJV). And on top of that, He also has "borne *our* griefs and carried *our* sorrows" (verse 4, NKJV).

Knowing that Jesus willingly accepted a "no" from God, despite the pain it involved, was a tremendous encouragement to me as I slowly released my grip on my dream for a pregnancy. But as inspiring as it was, Christ's example wasn't the only scriptural model that helped me come to spiritual closure. I didn't look for a biblical personality who made it through infertility successfully. I focused on someone who, like me, had an intense desire to do something good and honorable, but who, also like me, couldn't fulfill his dream because God said no.

I'm talking about David, the king of Israel. This man after God's own heart had a great desire to build a temple—"a house for the Name of the LORD [his] God" (1 Chronicles 22:7). But because he had fought in many wars and shed much blood, God would not allow him to construct the temple (verse 8). If you think about it, this really doesn't seem fair. After all, David wasn't waging war out of some sadistic need to destroy people—he was carrying out God's plan to defeat Israel's enemies. In a way, it was his obedience that kept him from building the temple.

I'm sure that David was extremely disappointed that he could not oversee this impressive construction project. He might have even been very upset about it at first. But he didn't dwell on it. He accepted God's decree, and he devoted his final years to making "extensive preparations" to ensure that his son, Solomon, would be able to build a temple for the Lord that would be "of great magnificence and fame and splendor in the sight of all the nations" (1 Chronicles 22:5).

Here's how he summarized his efforts in his final charge to Solomon:

> I have taken great pains to provide for the temple of the LORD a hundred thousand talents of gold, a million talents of silver, quantities of bronze and iron too great to be weighed, and wood and stone. And you may add to

them. You have many workmen: stonecutters, masons and carpenters, as well as men skilled in every kind of work in gold and silver, bronze and iron-craftsmen beyond number. Now begin the work, and the LORD be with you (1 Chronicles 22:14-16).

David didn't just organize the materials, however. The following verse reports that he also "ordered all the leaders of Israel to help his son Solomon" (verse 17). He did everything in his power to make sure the project was a success, no matter who completed it. He was more concerned about giving God glory than he was about adding an impressive accomplishment to his own résumé.

Instead of getting bitter, he made the best of a disappointing situation. He didn't try to forge ahead and build a temple on his own. He obeyed God, and his obedience allowed his son to construct a glorious temple. What a wonderful example for us to follow!

If you've been unable to conceive despite years of infertility treatment, God may be telling you that He has other plans for you. You may be tempted to deal with your disappointment by pouting and grumbling and being miserable. If you want to experience peace and joy in your life, however, you need to accept His will and find a way to make the best of it. Rather than mourning all you've lost, perhaps you need to make Philippians 3:13-14 your new motto: "One thing I do: Forgetting what is behind and straining toward what is ahead, I press on toward the goal to win the prize for which God has called me heavenward in Christ Jesus."

What Next?

Once you make the decision to stop trying to get pregnant, you are faced with an even bigger decision: what "pressing on toward the goal" should look like for your family. After directing all your energy toward achieving one goal for so long, it can be difficult to switch gears. But it can be done.

You already know the options—adoption, foster-parenting, or living without children (a "family of two," as one author put it[2]). I'm not going to tell you which one is right for you. That's for you and your spouse to decide. Friends, relatives, and acquaintances will be quick to offer their opinions, but don't base your decisions on what they have to say, especially if it's negative. You are the one who will have to live with your choice for the rest of your life, not them. So you need to do whatever it takes to ensure that you make the correct decision. That might involve spending time with adoptive couples and foster parents, talking to infertile people who chose not to adopt, researching the pros and cons of each option, and seeking godly counsel from trusted spiritual mentors.

When you talk to other people who have been where you are, ask them to be as honest and upfront as possible. Why did they do what they did? What (if anything) do they regret about the path they took? What would they do differently if they had to do it all over again? How did they know it was the right route for them? What should you consider as you think through all your options? In addition to asking questions, observe how they relate to each other as husband and wife, how they relate to their children (if they have any), and if they appear to be content and at peace. When you combine these observations with what they say, you'll have a more complete idea of whether or not their advice and counsel about this matter is reliable and credible.

You may wonder if you can really know if God's plan for you includes adoption. Such ambiguity is understandable—taking another person's child into your heart and home is a huge step. But I truly believe that if you have been praying for God's will to be done regarding your family, you will know whether or not you are supposed to adopt. Long before you even thought about relinquishing your dream to have biological children, God was already at work in your heart, preparing it for whatever He wants you to do next. And if that includes adoption, you'll know it.

When I was growing up—and even in the early years of my marriage—I never thought about adoption. I knew people who were adopted, and I didn't have anything against it. But I just never thought it was something I would want or need to do. As Randy and I prayed for a baby, however, something deep within me started to change. I can't remember a particular time when I decided that adoption would be okay for me, or that I would

---

There is life after infertility, even though you might doubt it right now.

---

actually *like* to adopt. As our chances of becoming pregnant grew slimmer and slimmer, we just started talking about adopting as if it had been a part of our plan all along.

After going through several surgeries and completing our previously agreed-upon infertility treatment, Randy and I were even more firmly convinced that we wanted children. It was as if God took our natural desire for a family and expanded it to cover children who weren't related to us by blood, but whom we could love just as much as any child who was made up of our genetic material. I can't tell you how or when this happened. I just know that it did happen. Moving forward with adoption was as natural for us as is getting pregnant for couples who don't have infertility problems. It just felt right.

Your experience may not mirror ours exactly. But the process for deciding upon your next step could be similar. The key, once again, lies in praying for God's will to be done and being willing to release all your expectations and desires completely to Him, trusting that He knows what is best for your life. Only when you relinquish your own agenda can you be confident you will be able to hear God's voice about what you are to do next. If you're still holding on to your old dreams or pouting because they were not fulfilled, you will not have the objectivity you need to make critical decisions about the future of your family.

If God leads you to adopt, you may move straight from infertility treatment into adoption (as we did). Or you might need to give yourself some time to recuperate emotionally and financially. Remember, the same rules of stewardship you followed when you were coming up with an infertility treatment strategy also apply in this situation. Going into debt, even if it's for a worthy cause such as domestic or international adoption, is never a good idea.

There's always the possibility that God may call you to invest your lives in people outside your immediate family, either through work or ministry endeavors, rather than pursue adoption. I have a couple of friends who chose this route, and they are some of the most loving, empathetic, and fulfilled people I know.

If you truly believe this is the path God wants you to take, don't ever feel as if you have to make excuses for it or let anyone think that you have selected a less spiritual option than someone who chose adoption. Just be prepared for an onslaught of questions. You may even meet with criticism from other Christians who don't understand your choice. Some people will think you're selfish. Others will feel sorry for you because you're missing out on all the wonderful blessings that accompany parenthood. God can use you just as much—if not more so—as a childless couple or individual than He could if you had children, so you'll just have to grow an extra layer of skin to deflect any undeserved criticism you may receive.

The Alternate Ending

You will be truly content with the family option that you choose only if you first make a conscious decision to let go of your dream of having biological children. Letting go doesn't mean that God can't or won't surprise you with an unexpected pregnancy somewhere down the road. But it does mean that you aren't planning your life around the possibility that such a miracle might occur.

Holding on leads to bitterness and misery. But letting go opens the door to peace and acceptance. And I can testify that the latter is definitely better than the former.

When we released our dream of getting pregnant, God replaced it with a new dream—to adopt a baby girl from China. Looking back, I can honestly say that our experience has been (as Randy once described it) like a movie with an alternate ending—one that turned out to be even better than the original conclusion.

That's what happens when you relinquish your dreams to the One who drew up the plans for your life—"plans to prosper you and not to harm you, plans to give you hope and a future" (Jeremiah 29:11).

TWELVE

Count Your Blessings

～～～

*A*s you navigate the bumpy road of infertility, you will no doubt come across other Christians who pity you because you haven't been able to have your "own" children or wonder how a person without biological children can have even an ounce of meaning and fulfillment in his or her life.

If you were to ask these people to justify their opinions biblically, most would probably point to Psalm 127:3-5. This is a familiar passage, one that can send fiery darts of pain through the heart of an infertile couple. "Sons are a heritage from the LORD, children a reward from him," it says. "Like arrows in the hands of a warrior are sons born in one's youth. Blessed is the man whose quiver is full of them" (Psalm 127:2-5).

I agree that children are wonderful blessings. If they were not, infertility wouldn't be nearly as hard as it is. I also understand why people with children might count them among the greatest blessings in their lives. But to suggest that people without children (married or not) are somehow missing out on the ultimate blessing is both narrow-minded and unbiblical. The Scriptures (especially Psalms and Proverbs) list dozens of other sources of

God's blessing. And nearly all of these have to do with a person's heart and relationship to God and others, rather than her ability to reproduce her own genetic material.

For example, you are blessed when you refrain from walking in the "counsel of the wicked" or standing "in the way of sinners" or sitting "in the seat of mockers" (Psalm 1:1). You're blessed when you delight in the law of the Lord and meditate on it around the clock (Psalm 1:2). You are blessed if your "transgressions are forgiven" and your "sins are covered" (Psalm 32:1). You're blessed when you take refuge in the Lord (Psalm 34:8), when you make the Lord your trust (Psalm 40:4), when you have regard for the weak (Psalm 41:1), when you learn to acclaim the Lord and walk in His presence (Psalm 89:15), when you seek Him with all your heart (Psalm 119:2), when you maintain justice, and when you "constantly do what is right" (Psalm 106:3).

You're blessed when you are kind to the needy (Proverbs 14:21), when you are generous to the poor (Proverbs 22:9), when you are faithful (Proverbs 28:20), when you honor the Sabbath (Isaiah 56:3), when you are disciplined by God (Psalm 94:12), when you find wisdom (Proverbs 3:13), when you serve others (John 13:11-17), when you fear the Lord continually (Proverbs 28:14), when you read the book of Revelation and take its message to heart (Revelation 1:3-4), and when you actively watch for the return of Jesus Christ (Revelation 16:14-15).

Blessing Through Difficulty

The New Testament also reveals that great blessing often flows out of suffering and pain. Matthew 5:3-12 makes a convincing case for this:

> Blessed are the poor in spirit,
>   for theirs is the kingdom of heaven.
> Blessed are those who mourn,
>   for they will be comforted.

Blessed are the meek,
  for they will inherit the earth.
Blessed are those who hunger and thirst for
  righteousness,
  for they will be filled.
Blessed are the merciful,
  for they will be shown mercy.
Blessed are the pure in heart,
  for they will see God.
Blessed are the peacemakers,
  for they will be called sons of God.
Blessed are those who are persecuted because of
  righteousness,
  for theirs is the kingdom of heaven.

Blessed are you when people insult you, persecute you and falsely say all kinds of evil against you because of me. Rejoice and be glad, because great is your reward in heaven, for in the same way they persecuted the prophets who were before you.

Notice that this passage says nothing about having children. Like most of the blessings delineated in the Old Testament, all the blessings here are a direct result of Christlike behavior, not familial relationships.

God may not have blessed you with biological children yet. And He may never choose to do so. But regardless of whether you ever have a successful pregnancy, you have many other wonderful opportunities to receive His blessing, most of which can have eternal impact. In the meantime, you can either bemoan the fact that you're missing out on the blessing of children (either temporarily or permanently), or you can actively seek out ways to grow in purity and godliness, serve others, and develop wisdom. The choice is yours.

Other Blessings

In addition to having access to all these spiritual blessings, you also have been given an abundance of material and relational blessings in your life. You may feel cursed because of your infertility, but if you turn your attention away from that reality for a minute and start reviewing all the other good things in your life, you'll quickly realize that you have much for which to be joyful.

My own list includes a vibrant marriage to a devoted husband, close relationships with my parents and siblings, a lovely (though not extravagant) home, wonderful friends, a great church, the opportunity to write and share my life experiences with other hurting people, and good health (despite my continuing battle with endometriosis, I'm rarely sick and have no other recurring physical problems). Your list (and I encourage you to put it on paper) may look very different. But if you give it some thought, I'm sure you'll come to find out that you are far more blessed than you may have realized.

I don't want to forget what it feels like to be totally dependent on God.

Helen Keller once said, "When one door of happiness closes, another opens. But often we spend so much time looking at the closed doors that we cannot see the doors that have opened for us. We must find all these doors, and, if we do, we will make ourselves and our lives as beautiful as God intended."[1]

The door that leads to the blessing of biological children might be closing quickly for you. Or it might already be tightly shut. Either way, you need to start looking for other doors that God is preparing for you. Some of these may lead to alternative plans for building your family, while others might lead you down a different career path or open to exciting new ministry opportunities. As long as you're willing to set aside your own expectations for your life and commit to following God's plan wholeheartedly, you will be able to find joy and peace beyond whatever door eventually opens to you.

As we've learned, giving birth to biological children is not the loftiest goal you can aspire to. Neither is the inability to have children the end of the world. Jesus said, "I have come that they might have life, and have it to the full" (John 10:10). As a Christian, you are able to have a full life because of Jesus and His work in you and through you, not because of the number of offspring you produce. It is only by focusing on His character, His sovereignty, His love, and His promises that you can ever hope to enjoy all the other blessings He has so generously bestowed upon you.

You may find this hard to believe, but eventually, you may even come to view your infertility as a blessing. You might want to put it out of your mind completely right now, but there may come a day when memories of your infertility journey elicit feelings of thankfulness, rather than pain. There may come a day when, instead of making you cry, those emotional flashbacks we talked about earlier will prompt you to fall on your knees in humble worship.

I realize that this might sound a bit radical, even completely crazy. But I know it can happen, because it has happened to me. Let me explain.

As much as I hate to stumble across those painful reminders of my infertility journey, and as frustrating as it is to deal with bursts of emotion that seem to come out of nowhere, I don't want them to stop. Why, you ask? The answer is simple.

I don't *want* to forget.

I don't want to forget what it feels like to be totally dependent on God. I don't want to forget all the valuable lessons I learned as

I waited for a baby—lessons about myself, about God, about my marriage, about the suffering of others. I don't want to forget the spiritual growth that occurred in my life as a result of this trial.

The good news—as odd as it might sound—is that God won't let me forget. I'm reminded every month as I cope with varying amounts of pain from my endometriosis. As I steel myself for the inevitable, I always end up meditating upon the same passage of Scripture. "You created my inmost being; you knit me together in my mother's womb," I pray, gaining strength with each passing word.

> *I praise you because I am fearfully and wonderfully*
> *   made;*
> *   your works are wonderful,*
> *   I know that full well.*
> *My frame was not hidden from you*
> *   when I was made in the secret place.*
> *When I was woven together in the depths of the earth,*
> *   your eyes saw my unformed body.*
> *All the days ordained for me*
> *   were written in your book*
> *   before one of them came to be.*
> *   —Psalm 139:12-16*

As these marvelous truths permeate my spirit and restore my soul, I'm reminded of another biblical blessing that has nothing to do with fertility and everything to do with trusting God in the midst of suffering: "Blessed is the man who perseveres under trial, because when he has stood the test, he will receive the crown of life that God has promised to those who love him" (James 1:12).

The blessings just don't get any better than that.

The Ripples Continue

~~~~~~

*W*hen Randy and I were trying to get pregnant, I often wondered if the peace I was experiencing as a result of our prayers would remain once we had a child. Would this divine serenity that "transcends understanding" continue to guide my heart and mind as I raised my children? Or would my old nemesis of worry start rearing its ugly head again and again? And what if I were diagnosed with cancer or suffered some other personal tragedy? Would the peace still be there, or was it merely temporary?

I can't answer all those questions with 100-percent certainty because I can't see into the future. But I do know this: I am a different person today than I was five years ago when we embarked on our quest for conception. My faith, then practically nonexistent and certainly untested, is exponentially stronger. As I explained in chapter five, I no longer struggle with worry like I used to. And the peace that God gave me as Randy and I maneuvered through the sometimes-rough waters of infertility has continued to protect me as we navigate the often-frustrating seas of international adoption.

Through it all, I've come to realize that the peace that came through infertility was not specific to infertility. Rather, it was the result of a deepening trust in and dependence on our loving heavenly Father. It is an everlasting peace, one that affects every area of my life.

Let me give you a few examples. When terrorists struck our country on September 11, 2001, I was as shocked and horrified as any other American. But even as my heart grieved for the thousands of people who lost loved ones in the tragedies, I was experiencing a tranquility about the whole situation that was completely new to me. Before, I would have been consumed by fear, worry, and anxiety. Instead, as I clung to my belief in God's sovereignty, I was comforted by the knowledge that His purposes would ultimately prevail, no matter what other horrors the evildoers of this world might carry out.

Several months after September 11, my father began having a perplexing set of symptoms that included occasional disorientation, temporary memory loss, and a fainting spell. Needless to say, this was a somewhat scary and uncertain time for my family. When a 68-year-old man experiences such troubles, scenarios such as heart problems, brain tumors, and Alzheimer's disease aren't just passing worries—they're distinct possibilities.

But despite the potential for such grave outcomes, I once again felt that indescribable peace that only comes from above. I didn't welcome the thought that my dad might die. And I especially didn't want to think about the fact that if he passed away soon, he wouldn't get to meet the daughter Randy and I were in the process of adopting. But because of what I had learned as I tried to get pregnant, I was certain that God was in control, and that whatever would happen to my father was part of His good and perfect plan. Such knowledge encouraged my heart as we waited for test results that eventually revealed that my dad was suffering from a correctable form of mild epilepsy.

My point in telling you these stories is simple. If these events had occurred prior to my infertility journey, I would have responded to each one by becoming the world's biggest basket case. But because of the heavenly peace that had infiltrated my life as Randy and I attempted to conceive, I was able to face each of these situations with courage and an extraordinary sense of calmness. I didn't respond this way because I possessed some astounding amount of faith or a massive quantity of strength. My response was solely and completely due to the peace of God that relentlessly guarded my heart and mind.

It can be that way for you, too, if you take what I've written in this book to heart. Allow God to use your struggles with infertility—whether temporary or permanent—as a means to make you more like Him. The peace that comes through infertility will continue to protect your soul long after you shut the door on further treatment or complete a successful pregnancy. It will remain with you as you ascend to life's most magnificent mountaintops, as well as when you pass through the darkest valleys. You can be sure of this because the Source of that peace has promised never to leave you nor forsake you (Hebrews 13:5).

That's cause enough to rejoice, but it gets even better. As the peace that surpasses understanding begins to soothe your upset stomach, erase the worry lines on your forehead, and eliminate the tightness at the base of your neck, other people will be able to see that there is something dramatically different about you.

In our frenetic, anxiety-ridden world, peace-filled individuals are the exception, not the norm (even in Christian circles). And if you're demonstrating peace in the midst of a difficult trial such as infertility, your words, actions, and countenance can't help but become tremendous testimonies of God's love and faithfulness. As I often say, people might attempt to dispute the facts of Christianity, but they can't argue with a changed life. The responsibility, then, is on you to "always be prepared to give an answer to everyone who asks you to give the reason for the hope that you have" (1 Peter 3:15).

When Randy and I decided to "start a family," I had no idea what the coming years would hold for me. (It's a good thing, too—had I known, I might not have had the fortitude to keep going.) Even now, as I try to imagine what might lie ahead, the picture is fuzzy at best. But that's okay. God has been faithful to me in the past, and He will continue to be faithful in the future. He can't help it—it's part of His character.

> *The peace that comes through infertility will continue to protect your soul long after you shut the door on further treatment or complete a successful pregnancy.*

This understanding allows me to be, as Oswald Chambers once wrote, "certain in my uncertainty." Here's how Chambers explained this amazingly liberating concept:

> Our natural inclination is to be so precise—trying always to forecast accurately what will happen next—that we look upon uncertainty as a bad thing….The nature of the spiritual life is that we are certain in our uncertainty….Certainty is the mark of the commonsense life—gracious uncertainty is the mark of the spiritual life. To be certain of God means that we are uncertain in all our ways, not knowing what tomorrow may bring. This is generally expressed

with a sigh of sadness, but it should be an expression of breathless expectation. We are uncertain of the next step, but we are certain of God. As soon as we abandon ourselves to God and do the task He has placed closest to us, He begins to fill our lives with surprises.[1]

Such surprises may not have chubby cheeks and baby soft skin. They may even be unpleasant at times. But because they come from God, they will always be for our good. Always.

Your efforts to conceive may conclude with the happy surprise ending every infertile couple dreams of. Or they might grind to a halt as you face the more sobering reality that God may have other plans for your family. Whatever the case, my desire for you is this: "I pray that the eyes of your heart may be enlightened, so that you may know what is the hope of His calling, what are the riches of the glory of His inheritance in the saints, and what is the surpassing greatness of His power toward us who believe" (Ephesians 1:18-19, NASB).

Therein lies true peace—in the midst of infertility, and beyond.

When Someone You Love Is Infertile

⁓≈⁓

When I began thinking about writing a book on infertility, one of my primary goals was to help people cope with all the advice and "encouragement" that friends, loved ones, and even total strangers offer about the best ways to get pregnant, adoption, God's will, and other such topics. I was fielding a lot of these questions and comments myself. And I was becoming increasingly frustrated by the lack of sensitivity so many otherwise kindhearted people demonstrated as they tried to comfort me. As a result, I also wanted to give all these well-meaning folks some guidance about how to help an infertile friend, as well as how not to help.

The years passed, and I began to get used to the idea that my husband, Randy, and I would probably never have biological children. During this time the focus of my message began to shift. As I dealt with challenging lessons about acceptance, contentment, and trust, I started to sense a need for a resource that helps people who are having trouble conceiving learn how they can experience true peace in the midst of their struggle. Gradually,

God's sovereignty and peace became the driving force behind this project, as opposed to other people and the things they say and do.

I didn't forget my original intention, however. As my book took shape, I purposely included a chapter designed to help infertile people deal with unsolicited advice and encouragement. I also decided to add a separate appendix for you—the friends and family members of people dealing with infertility—because the way you respond to your loved ones' fertility problems can either enhance or decrease the level of peace they're feeling as they try to make it through this unwelcome season of life.

I want you to be able to read this and immediately understand what helps and what hinders, what works and what hurts, and what encourages versus what simply annoys. In other words, I plan to give you an up-close-and-personal look at how what you say and do affects me as an infertile person. I'm not going to beat around the bush because that would be a waste of your time and my energy. Rather, I'm going to tell you what your infertile friends and relatives might tell you if you asked them to be brutally honest about what you can do to make their journey a little easier.

Because you're reading this, I know you want to help your loved one who is having difficulty getting pregnant. But no matter how compassionate or caring you might be, you need to realize that you will never fully understand what it's like to experience infertility unless you have experienced it yourself. The lack of a child is the most obvious sign of infertility. But actually it affects nearly every aspect of a person's life, from her health, marriage, and self-image to her view of the future, her finances, and her relationship with God. There's just no way you can be aware of all that, especially because what is bothering someone one day might be completely forgotten the next. But that's okay. If they're even remotely reasonable, people who are struggling to conceive don't expect you to know exactly what they're going through—they just want you to care for them and love them without judging them or telling them what to do.

That said, let's delve into a few specific examples of what does *not* work if you're trying to encourage me about my infertility.

I Don't Want to Hear...

Medical Advice and Fertility Folklore

I don't care how many graduate degrees you've earned or how many articles about infertility you've read. If you're not a gynecologist or a reproductive endocrinologist, please don't give me advice about how to get pregnant. Don't tell me to relax, or to remain on my back for an hour after intercourse, or to take a nice vacation, or to try this herbal remedy or that nutritional supplement. Whatever you recommend will likely have no effect on the cause of my infertility.

Along the same lines, please don't offer unsolicited opinions—pro or con—about infertility procedures such as in vitro fertilization, artificial insemination, and so on. Such choices are between me, my spouse, and God. Unless I specifically ask for counsel from you, I really don't need to know what you think about these sensitive issues.

Pat Spiritual Answers

Chances are, when you talk to me about my infertility, you don't know exactly what to say. But whatever you do, stay away from pat spiritual answers. Don't try to tie things up for me in a neat little box. It just doesn't work. Infertility is messy. Every single case is different. So don't tell me that you just know God is going to give me a baby, that it's God's will for me to get pregnant, or that you're sure everything will work out. You have no way of knowing that. And don't tell me to pray harder, trust more, or have more faith. It's not that simple.

I know this might sound kind of odd, but please refrain from quoting familiar Bible verses to me. And I'd greatly appreciate it if you would bite your tongue when you're tempted to say something such as "If it's meant to be, it will happen" or "God is in control." It's not that I don't derive great comfort from biblical concepts such as God's sovereignty, but when you distill such awesome truths down to trite little nuggets of wisdom, you're more likely to annoy me than to help me.

Anecdotes About Other People

If I had a dollar for every infertility success story I've heard in the last few years, I'd probably have enough to take a very nice vacation. I don't mean to be rude, but I don't want to hear about your sister, cousin, or next-door neighbor who had severe endometriosis and now has three biological children. Nor do I want to hear about your friend or co-worker who tried to conceive for seven years, gave up, and is now expecting baby number two.

Those stories are wonderful, and I'm happy for those people. But this isn't about you and your stories, as hopeful as they are. It's about me and my life. You disregard my sadness when you rush to tell me all kinds of anecdotes about people you know. Just because it happened to them does not mean it will happen to me. It might, but it might not. For my own mental and emotional health, I have to deal with reality as it exists for me today. Although your anecdotes may be somewhat encouraging to people in the earliest stages of infertility, the longer the journey lasts, the less welcome they are.

You might think that such stories would stop coming once a couple decides to adopt, but I've found just the opposite to be true. If you've read the rest of this book, you know that I wrote it while my husband and I were in the process of adopting our first child, a baby girl from China. Nearly everyone we told about our adoption plans was very happy for us. But after asking us a few questions about the specifics, almost everyone had this bit of encouragement for us: "Just you wait. As soon as you get that baby home, you're going to get pregnant!" Such proclamations were nearly always followed by a glowing report about a friend, co-worker, or relative who had conceived after completing an adoption.

As someone whose chances of getting pregnant are practically nil, I can assure you that this was the last thing I wanted to hear when I told someone my happy news. The fact of the matter is, as I noted earlier in this book, only about 5 percent of women who adopt go on to get pregnant—5 percent![1] On top of that, many couples, including Randy and me, decide to adopt after most, if not all, of their hopes of conceiving are gone. We've closed the door to that possibility and are now moving on with our lives. So when you tell me stories about people who adopted and then got pregnant, you make it seem as if my adopted child will be some sort of temporary fix until the real blessing arrives. That is simply not the case.

The moral of the story is this: When people tell you they're having trouble getting pregnant, or when they tell you they've decided to adopt, don't try to encourage them by sharing infertility success stories with them. If you insist on doing this, all you'll do is detract from their pain or diminish their joy.

Negative Comments About Pregnancy, Childbirth, and Parenthood

If you're pregnant, you might think that you will make me feel better about my situation if you tell me how miserable you are, how difficult your last delivery was, or how long it took you to get back into shape after you had your last child. Such reverse psychology is not effective. I would gladly throw up every single morning if it meant that in seven or eight months, I would give birth to a healthy child. I would be thrilled to gain 30 extra pounds if it meant I could have a baby who looked like me or Randy. So please don't try to console me by pointing out all the "unpleasant" aspects of pregnancy that I'm missing out on.

Now it may be that you're complaining about being pregnant because you simply like to whine about how awful you feel, how tired you are, and how big you're getting. In other words, you're not doing it to make me feel better. You're just doing it to elicit sympathy. If that's the case, all I ask is that you practice a little consideration and keep those complaints to a minimum when I'm with you. I realize pregnancy can put a tremendous strain on a body, so I'm not saying a little griping isn't in order every now and then. But try to do it when I'm not around. It's hard for me to feel sorry for you when you are complaining about things I would love to be experiencing myself.

Solutions to the Problem of Childlessness

If I had to rank all the thoughtless things people say from most to least hurtful, the phrase, "You can always adopt" would be right up there at the top of the list. I know adoption sounds like a logical solution to the problem of childlessness. However, a glib comment like this fails to address all the painful questions and issues that not being able to conceive brings up in a person's life. As wonderful as it is, adoption does not automatically erase all the physical brokenness, theological confusion, and emotional distress that infertility causes.

The lack of a baby might be the most obvious ramification of my infertility. But it's not necessarily my most serious problem. In addition to an empty nursery, I'm also dealing with unmet expectations, the loss of dreams, health issues and physical pain, questions about God's will, doubts about my faith, and so on. Before I can ever hope to become a good adoptive parent, I need to begin the process of dealing with these deeper issues. Otherwise, my adopted child will never be more than what "you can always adopt" implies that she is—a consolation prize.

You also need to remember that adoption isn't for everyone. I know this might be difficult to understand, especially if you have several kids and know the joys that children can bring. But some couples, when confronted with the reality that they cannot have children, sense that God is leading them toward areas of service that may have nothing to do with diapers and formula. Of course, some couples don't adopt because either the husband or the wife is unwilling to expand their family that way. But you don't know any of this when you discover that someone can't have children and isn't planning to adopt. So it's best not to offer advice or encouragement about adoption unless you're asked for it.

Comments such as "Maybe God knows you wouldn't be a very good mother" or "Some people just aren't cut out to be parents" also can drive a stake straight through the heart of an infertile person. Thankfully, nobody has ever said anything like that to me. If someone had, my response might have landed me in jail. But I know that other people have been subjected to such statements, and that fact never ceases to boggle my mind. Why anyone would think that these remarks were even remotely helpful or encouraging is just beyond me.

Other Thoughtless Remarks

Before I move on to some positive ways that you can help me cope with my infertility, I need to mention a few other general "don'ts." First of all, if you have to precede anything you're about to say with "I know you've probably heard this a hundred times…"—*don't* say it. You're right. I probably have heard it a hundred times. And I have no desire to hear it again.

Also, if the sentence you're about to utter begins with the words "at least…" don't say it. "At least you still have each other" won't make me feel better about not having a baby. "At least you know you can get pregnant" won't lessen my grief at having a miscarriage. "At least you don't have cancer" won't prevent me from feeling as if my body is broken. I could go on all day, but surely you get the picture. Anything that follows the words "at least" only trivializes the pain and loss I'm experiencing due to my infertility.

Such comments never help. Hopefully, there will come a day when I am able to think of these things on my own and recognize that my life is complete and full of blessings even without a bio-logical child. But I need to get there on my own timetable.

As I said before, it's hard for someone who has not struggled with infertility to fully comprehend what a difficult issue it is, as well as how hurtful it is when people make insensitive remarks such as those I've just mentioned. If you're still a bit confused about what not to say, perhaps this will help. Think of a trial that you have experienced in your life—the death of a loved one, a serious illness, the infidelity of a spouse, a divorce, a financial struggle, or something similar. Do you remember how you felt when someone tried to console you with pious platitudes or pat answers? I'm sure you do. So here's the main point: Don't say anything to comfort me about my infertility that you would not have wanted someone to say to you when you were walking through your own difficulty. It's that simple.

How to Help

Now that we've covered everything I *don't* want you to say, you're probably wondering if there's anything you *can* do to help me deal with infertility. Fortunately, you can do much more than you may think. And you should. Life as a barren person can be very lonely—I'm somewhat of a misfit in a society that is so oriented around children. This is especially true in the church, where motherhood is considered to be one of life's most noble callings. I don't want you to feel sorry for me—but as I said before, I do want you to care.

So how should you start? Romans 12:15 spells it out: "Rejoice with those who rejoice; mourn with those who mourn." Notice that this verse says nothing about offering advice, passing judg-ment, providing words of wisdom, or asking nosy questions. The meaning of the second phrase of the verse is clear—you are to grieve with me when I'm sad. Nothing more, nothing less.

I'm reminded of what Job's three friends did first when they went to see him after he lost everything. "They sat on the ground with him for seven days and seven nights. No one said a word to him, because they saw how great his suffering was" (Job 2:13). Job's friends get a bad rap for what they did next—talk about falling flat on one's face in the encouragement department! But they did get it right at first. They just sat with Job and said nothing.

Many times, that is all I want from you. I just want you to sit with me and not say anything at all. I know that's hard to do. We're so programmed to provide solutions and answers. But in this case, there are no answers, at least not ones that are readily available. If you do feel compelled to say something, just tell me you're sorry about what I'm going through. Tell me that you can't imagine how I must feel. Tell me you have no idea how difficult infertility must be. Ask me if I want to talk about it. If I do, just listen.

Ask me how you can pray for me. Don't just assume that I want you to pray that I'll get pregnant. I may want you to do that. But I may have other needs too. I may need courage for a particular test. Or I may desire wisdom to make a decision about a particular treatment or procedure. I might want you to pray that God will give me the strength to accept His will, whatever that might be, or I might want you to ask God to give me opportunities to use my suffering to minister to others. You won't know any of this unless you ask.

Although women receive most of the attention when it comes to infertility, husbands have feelings too. Men are particularly guilty of making insensitive comments to other men about manhood, parenting, adoption, and other similar issues. Guys may not take such comments to heart as much as women do, but they still hurt.

Use what you learn from me in your conversations with other young couples. You never know whether someone you meet might be having trouble getting pregnant, so be aware of what you say. Never ask a married person, "Do you have a family?" Most people equate families with children—but a husband and a wife are just as much of a family as a couple with six kids. "How many children do you have?" also is a bad choice. "Do you have any children?" is much more sensitive. If the answer is no, don't ask why not. If I want you to know, I'll tell you—if not, just let it go. "Do you hope to have children someday?" is another acceptable inquiry. If I don't want to talk about it, I can give you a vague response. If I do, I can explain further.

While you should be cognizant of how what you say might affect me, I don't want you to feel as if you have to walk on eggshells around me. You were an important part of my life before I started experiencing infertility. Although life has sent us down different paths for now, I still value your friendship. I don't want to be the last to know that you're pregnant. I do want to be invited to baby showers and children's birthday parties. Don't be offended if I choose not to attend—if I'm feeling particularly vulnerable or sad that day, it might be best for me to stay home. But I do want to be included in the important things in your life, so please don't leave me out in your efforts to spare my feelings.

The bottom line is, although I may be unsure of how to verbalize it, I need your comfort, encouragement, and prayers now more than ever. Don't be afraid to ask me how you can help. And if you think about it, send me an encouraging note every now and then.

Above all else, remember this: Infertility is not a one-time ordeal. It's an ongoing struggle, one that can gradually wear away a person's confidence and hope. Your support might not be able to stop the erosion entirely, but it can certainly slow it down.

A Note to Pastors

～～～

Evangelical Christian churches are not the most welcoming places for infertile couples these days. I can't think of a nicer way to say it. They're just not. Much of church life revolves around children, parenting, and marriage, and adults who don't fit these demographics (barren couples and singles, for example) often feel very out of place. On top of that, some pastors—even those who deal primarily with young married couples—can be quite unknowledgeable about infertility and even somewhat insensitive to people who are having trouble getting pregnant or those who have made the decision to adopt or live without children.

It doesn't have to be that way, however. If you're a pastor, what you say and do—from the pulpit and elsewhere—can have a very positive impact on the spiritual health of the infertile members of your congregation. Your words and actions also can set an example for the other people in your church of how to treat fellow believers who are dealing with this issue.

One in ten Americans of childbearing age have fertility problems. This means that, if your ministry serves more than a couple hundred people, there's a good chance that at least a few of them fall into this category. You might not know who they are because many are unwilling to broadcast their personal struggles to the world. But that doesn't mean they're not out there, listening to what you say—and formulating their ideas about God and how He views them accordingly.

These people are hurting, and they're vulnerable. Because of that, your words have the power to increase their understanding of God's love and sovereignty or to push them away from the church altogether. I'm guessing you don't take that responsibility lightly, so here are a few tips that might help you minister to this segment of population a little better.

First, I want to encourage you to read this book very carefully—more than once, if possible. Don't just skim through the sections you think might apply. Study the whole thing so you can get a more complete picture of what a person who is having difficulty conceiving goes through emotionally and spiritually. If you have the opportunity to counsel couples who are struggling with infertility, make sure they have a proper understanding of God and His role in their lives, as explained in the second and third chapters.

In your preaching, be careful not to imply that children are God's ultimate blessing. Or that a woman is most fulfilled when she is married with children. If you ever offer special prayer for infertile couples (perhaps on Mother's Day), remember that contentment and acceptance of God's will are just as important, if not more so, than a positive pregnancy test. It may not be part of God's plan for every woman you pray for to become pregnant. However, the spiritual blessings that accompany peace and contentment are available to everyone who is open to receiving them.

Realize that unresolved infertility is a trial that never really goes away, even if a couple chooses to adopt. There may be ongoing health issues to contend with, and you never know when some event or date will trigger a memory that makes all the sadness come rushing back. Be sensitive to the fact that some women in your church—even ones in their forties or older—may choose to stay away on Mother's Day or other family-oriented holidays simply because they don't want to deal with all those painful emotions yet again. Your merciful response to such decisions is very important.

Perhaps you are part of a large church or a church that organizes small groups based on season of life (or age of children). If so, consider having a class for people who have been married for several years with no children. My church offered such a class when my husband and I were trying to get pregnant. It made a huge difference in our lives at that time. It wasn't the class itself that helped us as much as it was the opportunity to get to know other couples around our age who didn't have children. Before that time, we often felt all alone in a huge church full of families with children. The class helped us connect with people—some who were experiencing infertility and others who were not—who remain our friends to this day.

When you deal with the subject of miscarriage, either from the pulpit or in personal counseling, keep in mind that telling a grieving couple that their baby is in heaven isn't enough. That knowledge might provide some comfort, but it fails to address all the other painful issues associated with pregnancy loss. This is particularly true if the miscarriage comes after several years of infertility. Or if it is not the first miscarriage the couple has suffered. In such cases, couples are likely to wonder why God allowed them to get pregnant in the first place if He were just going to let the baby die. And that's only one example of the type of anguished questions a miscarriage precipitates. Your counsel in these situations may begin with assurances of the baby's eternal home, but if it doesn't eventually lead the grieving couples to a deeper understanding of God's sovereignty and providence, it won't help much.

Finally, consider adding infertility to the list of topics you cover in marriage counseling. You probably already ask engaged couples to talk about how many kids they want and how they plan to approach child-rearing. But it would also be helpful to encourage couples to think about how they might react if one or both was diagnosed with a fertility problem at some point. Nobody plans to be infertile. But if couples go into marriage with the understanding that it might be a problem, perhaps they won't be so blindsided by it if they start having trouble getting pregnant someday.

I'm sure there are many other ways that you can reach out to the infertile couples in your congregation. The key is to remember that they're out there, even though they may not make their presence known. And now, perhaps more than any other time in their lives, they need to know that their spiritual leaders accept them, care for them, and want them to experience abundant life—with or without children.

Appendix C

Recommended Reading

It would be impossible for me to list every book and Web site that might inform, comfort, or encourage you as you cope with the daily realities of infertility. That said, I would still like to mention at least a few resources that have helped me work through the medical, emotional, and spiritual issues relating to my inability to conceive.

For comprehensive information about infertility, including diagnosis and treatment options:

- *Experiencing Infertility* by Debby Peoples and Harriette Rovner Ferguson (W.W. Norton & Co. Inc., 1998)
- www.resolve.org, the Web site for RESOLVE: The National Infertility Association
- www.asrm.org, the Web site for the American Society for Reproductive Medicine
- www.protectyourfertility.com, an educational site from the American Society for Reproductive Medicine

For a Christian perspective on diverse aspects of infertility, including the pros and cons of various assisted reproductive technologies:

- *When Empty Arms Become a Heavy Burden* by Sandra Glahn and William Cutrer, M.D. (Broadman & Holman Publishers, 1997)
- *The Ache for a Child* by Debra Bridwell (Victor Books, 1994)

For faith-based encouragement when you feel as if you're all alone:

- *Empty Womb, Aching Heart* by Marlo Schalesky (Bethany House Publishers, 2001)

For comfort and encouragement following a miscarriage:

- *Losing You Too Soon* by Bernadette Keaggy (Harvest House Publishers, 2002)

For biblically based analyses of the ethical issues pertaining to infertility treatment options:

- www.cmdahome.org, the Web site for the Christian Medical Association (search for keyword "infertility")
- *Without Moral Limits: Women, Reproduction and Medical Technology* by Debra Evans (Crossway Books, 2000)

For a greater understanding of God's sovereignty and its role in your life:

- *The Mystery of God's Will* by Charles R. Swindoll (Word Publishing, 1999)
- *The Hand of God: Finding His Care in All Circumstances* by Alistair Begg (Moody Press, 1999)

When you're trying to make sense out of suffering:

- *Where Is God When It Hurts?* by Philip Yancey (Zondervan, 2001)
- *Disappointment with God* by Philip Yancey (Zondervan, 1997)
- *When God Doesn't Make Sense* by James Dobson (Tyndale House Publishers, Inc., 1993)
- *When God Weeps: Why Our Sufferings Matter to the Almighty* by Joni Eareckson Tada and Steve Estes (Zondervan Publishing House, 1997)

A daily devotional book to encourage you in your journey:

- *Diamonds in the Dust* by Joni Eareckson Tada (Zondervan Publishing House, 1993)

For instruction about the spiritual discipline of prayer and fasting:

- *The Power of Prayer and Fasting* by Ronnie W. Floyd (Broadman & Holman Publishers, 1997)

If you're thinking about expanding your family through adoption:

- *Adopting After Infertility* by Patricia Irwin Johnston (Perspectives Press, 1992)

For a fun diversion from all the infertility information:

- The Chronicles of Narnia by C.S. Lewis (HarperCollins Publishers, 1982)

Finally, for a powerful story that will help you put your own trials into perspective:

- *Safely Home* by Randy Alcorn (Tyndale House Publishers, 2001)

Notes

Chapter 1 — Why Peace Is Elusive

1. According to the American Society for Reproductive Medicine's Web site (<www.asrm.org/Patients/faqs.html#Q1:>), "infertility affects about 6.1 million people in the U.S.—about 10 percent of the reproductive age population."

2. According to RESOLVE and the American Society for Reproductive Medicine, infertility is unexplained in about 20 percent of cases. (See "Frequently asked questions about infertility" [<http://www.asrm.org/Patients/faqs.html#Q1:>] and "Infertility myths and facts" [<http://www.resolve.org/getstart/mythfact.shtml>].)

Chapter 2 — A Solid Starting Point

1. James Dobson, *When God Doesn't Make Sense* (Wheaton, IL: Tyndale House Publishers, Inc., 1993), pp. 14-15.

2. Charles R. Swindoll, *The Mystery of God's Will* (Nashville, TN: Word Publishing, 1999), p. 17.

Chapter 3 — His Ways Are Not Our Ways

1. Charles R. Swindoll, *The Mystery of God's Will* (Nashville, TN: Word Publishing, 1999), p. 87.

2. Frederick Buechner, as quoted in Philip Yancey, *Soul Survivor* (New York: Doubleday, 2001), p. 255.

3. See <www.resolve.org/main/national/trying/preserving/preserving1.jsp? name=trying&tag=preserving>.

4. Sandra Glahn and William Cutrer, M.D., *When Empty Arms Become a Heavy Burden* (Nashville, TN: Broadman & Holman Publishers, 1997), p. 114.

5. Swindoll, pp. 91-92.

6. Steven Curtis Chapman, "God Is God." © Peach Hill Songs 2/Sparrow Song. All Rights Reserved. Used By Permission.

7. Glahn and Cutrer, p. 128.

8. Michael Phillips, *Heathersleigh Homecoming* (Minneapolis, MN: Bethany House Publishers, 1999), pp. 142-143. Used with permission from *Heathersleigh Homecoming* by Michael Phillips © 1999 Bethany House Publishers. All Rights Reserved.

Chapter 4—How to Pray

1. Lois Flowers, *Women, Faith, and Work* (Nashville, TN: Word Publishing, 2001), p. 37.

2. Lois Flowers, "Shirley Forbes Thomas: When the Going Gets Tough," *Arkansas Democrat-Gazette*, November 18, 2001, p. 4D.

Chapter 6—Avoiding the Comparison Trap

1. C.S. Lewis, *The Horse and His Boy* (New York: HarperCollins Publishers, 1982), pp. 164-165.

Chapter 7—Thick Skin, Soft Heart

1. Debby Peoples, MSW, and Harriette Rovner Ferguson, CSW, *Experiencing Infertility* (New York: W.W. Norton & Co. Inc., 1998), p. 61.

Chapter 8—A Slightly Different Approach to Infertility Treatment

1. Debra Evans, *Without Moral Limits* (Wheaton, IL: Crossway Books, 2000), p. 94.

2. Sandra Glahn and William Cutrer, M.D., *When Empty Arms Become a Heavy Burden* (Nashville, TN: Broadman & Holman Publishers, 1997), p. 147.

3. Debra Bridwell, *The Ache for a Child* (Wheaton, IL: Victor Books, 1994), p. 291.

Chapter 9—Joining God

1. Marlo Schalesky, *Empty Womb, Aching Heart* (Bloomington, MN: Bethany House Publishers, 2001), pp. 143-144.
2. Debby Peoples, MSW, and Harriette Rovner Ferguson, CSW, *Experiencing Infertility* (New York: W.W. Norton & Co. Inc., 1998), p. 94.
3. Sandra Glahn and William Cutrer, M.D., *When Empty Arms Become a Heavy Burden* (Nashville, TN: Broadman & Holman Publishers, 1997), p. 150.
4. Charles R. Swindoll, *The Mystery of God's Will* (Nashville, TN: Word Publishing, 1999), p. 108.

Chapter 11—Letting Go of the Dream

1. This citation was taken from the RESOLVE Web site (www.resolve.org) in May 2002. In response to an e-mail inquiry for more information, RESOLVE spokeswoman Gina Cella provided the following statistics: 43 percent of infertile couples seek treatment. Of that group, 65 percent succeed in having a healthy baby. (This information was received via e-mail on June 17, 2002.)
2. Debra Bridwell, *The Ache for a Child* (Wheaton, IL: Victor Books, 1994), p. 262.

Chapter 12—Count Your Blessings

1. Patricia Irwin Johnston, *Adopting After Infertility* (Indianapolis, IN: Perspectives Press, 1992), p. 70.

Afterword—The Ripples Continue

1. Oswald Chambers, *My Utmost for His Highest: An Updated Version in Today's Language*, James G. Reimann, ed. (Grand Rapids, MI: Discovery House Publishers, 1992), April 29.

Appendix A—When Someone You Love Is Infertile

1. Debby Peoples, MSW, and Harriette Rovner Ferguson, CSW, *Experiencing Infertility* (New York: W.W. Norton & Co., Inc., 1998), p. 61.

Finding Hope Again...

Five months into her first pregnancy, Bernadette Keaggy gave birth to three beautiful sons. Tragically, they were stillborn. And over a period of years, Bernadette and her husband dealt with the pain of losing two more babies.

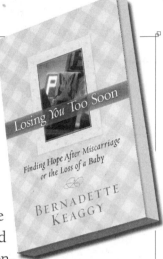

In *Losing You Too Soon,* Bernadette writes with honesty, compassion, and ultimately hope about the hurt and confusion she experienced and the effect this loss had on her self-esteem, her marriage, and her relationship with God. Her story doesn't offer simple solutions, but shows how to find the strength and courage to go on. You'll also find...

- practical advice for dealing with the loss of a baby
- important medical insights on premature birth and miscarriages
- the hope that comes from God's strength and comfort

Grieving couples know how hard it is to find someone who can truly understand what they are going through. For such readers, or those who seek to comfort them, this deeply moving book will be a source of profound encouragement and a reminder that God promises grace and hope in the midst of even the deepest pain.